T0106359

Fostering lifelong learning through student driven school and community activities

Developing the Leaders of Tomorrow Through Personal Growth Initiatives

Tina Bengermino

AuthorHouse™
1663 Liberty Drive
Bloomington, IN 47403
www.authorhouse.com
Phone: 1-800-839-8640

First published by AuthorHouse 12/2/2009

ISBN: 978-1-4490-5013-9 (sc)

Printed in the United States of America
Bloomington, Indiana

This book is printed on acid-free paper.

Table of Contents

Preface

I have written this book to introduce and promote *Personal Growth Initiatives* for students of all ages. If you are reading this because you are interested in or are currently implementing programs involving community service, volunteerism or service learning, I hope to convince you of the value of shifting to a Personal Growth Initiative Program. This book intends to guide your existing and new programs with effective ideas and materials.

Who am I? I am currently a middle and high school Health Education teacher in Fairfield, Connecticut. Prior to my shift into Health Education, I had been an elementary Physical Education teacher for seventeen years. I have a unique opportunity and pleasure to work with students from kindergarten through twelfth grade each year. During the year, I teach and coach at the middle and high school levels and in the summer I work with elementary students. So I am in touch with children at all levels of development which I feel not only keeps me young (well at least in mind- if not body) but also qualifies me to offer learning modifications to meet the needs of a variety of ages and ability levels.

My teaching philosophy and the thinking behind writing this book is basically that students should be encouraged to take healthy risks, to want to go beyond their comfort zone and be given the opportunity to practice doing so. I know many professionals share my sentiments but haven't seen a way to make it happen. This book, I believe, will provide not only the educational justification for such programs but also usable materials and guidelines that can be easily modified to your situation, wants and needs.

Introduction

After seventeen years of teaching elementary physical education, my first classroom position was as a health education teacher at Fairfield Woods Middle School in Fairfield Connecticut. The health education department in my town was, and still is, highly regarded statewide and often on the cutting edge of what was happening nationally in our profession. So, it was my good fortune to work with very dedicated and dynamic colleagues.

Cathy Hamill, my co-worker, along with Lori Mediate, our town's Education Department Coordinator, had developed what they called *The 7 Habits of Highly Effective People Project.* Of course, I had a choice of whether or not to utilize this project with my students when I arrived on the scene, but I really liked the basic premise behind the project. At first, I followed the model they had created, which included students performing an activity and identifying any qualities associated with Steven Covey's book titled, The 7 Habits of Highly Effective People. I saw the value in the learning and enjoyed doing these activities with my classes. However, over the years and through a collaborative effort with my teaching partner, Cathy Hamill, we have modified and expanded the project to become an exemplary model for a meaningful personal growth experience for young adults.

Cathy Hamill began, as I did, in teaching Physical Education before coming teaching Health Education. I believe our common roots in Physical Education may have lead to our unique philosophies and teaching approaches in the classroom setting. This may be due to the fact that physical education has always been a skill-based field where students are asked to demonstrate their learning. So, when we both left the gymnasium, we kept our expectations that our students should be able to demonstrate the acquisition of knowledge and skills as well as be able to carry over their classroom learning into their daily lives. This project and many of our assessments are developed with that mind set.

Cathy and I have given workshops at Health Education state and regional conventions sharing our teaching philosophies, programs and activities with colleagues. Time after time, our workshops have been met with great interest and requests for more information and details about two specific programs. One of the programs is *called The Contract for a Healthy Life* and the other *the Seven Habits of Highly Effective People* to which I referred earlier. Cathy Hamill has written a dynamic and thorough book titled The Contract for a Healthy Life which outlines the program of the same name.

I planned to write an account of the *Seven Habits of Highly Effective People Project* and give guidelines and materials for colleagues to be able to put this worthwhile project into action, yet I chose to wait until after I had finished my coursework on my sixth-year degree. I am so glad that I did. During my coursework, I heard over and over again the call for educational change and approaches to help students be prepared for the demands of the "new world". As I studied theories, new approaches, and the research of the day, I was struck by how many of these theories and approaches we were already utilizing and addressing in our programs. My delay in writing this book was auspicious because my work and reflections during these courses lead to me making some philosophical and practical modifications and to create some new ways to better reach my students and help you with yours. I trust that my approach is not only innovative but will ultimately lead our students to be better prepared to be successful, productive and happy adults.

Through my coursework and feedback from professors and classmates, I came to the realization that my understanding and experience in the use of skill based personal growth programs might be unique and worth sharing.

Well, there you have it... this is my rationale for writing this book. I fervently believe that if you have never tried reaching kids through a project like this, you will be sold the first time you try. If you have previously done a service learning or goal setting type project with students, you will see how much more meaningful and worthwhile the approaches I outline in this book will be for you as the teacher and for your students, as well.

Part One:

Why Use a Personal Growth Initiative?

Chapter One: Volunteerism, Community Service and Service Learning Programs

" We make a living by what we do, but we make a life by what we give." ~ Winston Churchill

I open this book with a discussion of service learning, community service projects and volunteerism because *Personal Growth Initiatives* are a natural outgrowth of these movements. My work was not begun with that intention but as I researched I found links to be evident. Also, the program our students are involved in has been labeled by the less informed as "community service projects" so I hope to clarify the differences between all the terms and programs. I think the trend for more of any of these kinds of programs is very positive for our schools, communities and nation, but I hope to make evident how *Personal Growth Initiatives* offer the most meaningful educational and personal experience for students.

Service learning is not a new phenomenon; however the trend in educational settings is growing not only in participation but acceptance.

The National Center for Educational Statistics (NCES) found that between 1984 and 1997, the number of kindergarten through twelfth grade students involved in service-learning programs rose from nine hundred thousand to over twelve million and the proportion of high school students participating grew twenty three percent. In 2001, the N.C.E.S. reported that thirteen million school students were involved in service and service learning.

The organization *Learn and Serve America* awards grants to state education agencies, schools, nonprofit groups and institutions of higher learning to engage students in service activities linked to academic achievement and civic responsibility. In a 2005 report, they profess to have almost one and a half million participants who have served over a total of twenty five million hours.

These statistics are wonderful, right? However, it is hard to interpret all the studies and statistics because service learning is still evolving, so is its definition and associated vocabulary. For example, what's the difference between being involved in service and service learning? Experts and organizations have not agreed upon one formal definition and I suggest that it might be detrimental to do so. A common definition may be limiting. I feel every program should have flexibility to create its own definition and parameters to meet its needs. However, I do believe it is important to have common language and vocabulary to understand one another. So what is service learning? How does it differ from community service and volunteerism?

Community Service and Volunteerism

Firstly, **volunteerism** is defined as performing unpaid work for an organization or a cause and **community service** refers to service that a person performs for the benefit of his or her local community. The distinctions may be minimal and whether it is accurate or not, most of us use these terms interchangeably. The undeniable fact is that both volunteerism and community service have positive connotations and those who perform them are praised. I plan to make the case that there is a very strong distinction between service learning and volunteerism/community service, but that they may not be exclusive of one another. Also, advocates of service learning believe that students who engage in service learning programs are more likely to volunteer later in life.

I'm pleased to say that volunteerism is at an all time high in our country especially following the tragedy on 9/11. Nearly sixty-one million Americans volunteered in their communities in 2007, and over twenty six percent of Americans aged sixteen and older gave over eight billion hours worth of service to American communities, according to the Corporation for National and Community Service. Now in 2009 we see President Obama appearing on television promoting the need for all Americans to get involved in community service. Recently a bill was passed to increase the size and scope of AmeriCorps, the government's largest volunteer organization and the domestic equivalent of the Peace Corps. Schools have responded in kind by running school wide community service projects, offering after school community service clubs and requiring community service hours for graduation.

Community Service; like volunteerism, might be undertaken for altruistic reasons but a new trend is for it to be done as a requirement for achievement. I have heard many say it does not matter why kids are serving others; it is simply a good thing and in the long run they will learn to appreciate and value it. This might be true, I think that this approach is not enough- we can do better for our youth!

In my research, I found many school districts, universities and colleges where a certain number of hours of community service are required to graduate. Are these participants really developing genuine civic responsibility and/or altruism? I say very few are and I question whether altruism learned in this context will really carry over into future behaviors. I also suggest that due to forced involvement there exists minimal student motivation which must impact the intended outcome. In my town's high schools, our students do not have such requirements for graduation, but students must meet a set number of volunteer hours to be included in the National Honor Society. Some of these academically high achieving high school students volunteer at my middle school. They have admitted to me that they are only doing it because they have to and many even consider falsifying their records to satisfy the requirements due to an already overloaded schedule.

Learning is at the heart of the **service learning** experience.

Many high schools and higher learning institutions are shifting their graduation requirements from volunteer and community service requirements to include involvement in service learning programs. One reason cited has been the component of service learning programs that requires students to demonstrate that their work has contributed to their education. And that's the clear distinction between volunteerism, community service and service learning. Learning is at the heart of the service learning experience.

The report "Learning in Deed: The Power of Service-Learning for American Schools (2001- the National Commission on Service-Learning) incorporated what it saw as the most essential features common to service learning programs across the country into this definition: **"Service Learning is different from volunteerism in that it is 'a teaching and learning approach that integrates community service with academic study to enrich learning, teach civic responsibility, and strengthen communities"(page 6).**

Again there is no one accepted definition. I believe the definition of service learning should be one that can be altered to fit differing needs and situations. This fact, of course, leads to differences among the experts as well. A definition that I especially liked and I feel readily conforms to various settings, can be found in Cathryne Berger Kaye's book, <u>The Complete Guide to Service Learning</u>. She writes..."**Service Learning can be defined as a teaching method where guided or classroom learning is deepened through service to others in a process that provides structured time for reflection on the service experience and demonstration of the skills and knowledge required**."

To get a slightly different view of how service learning is interpreted, I offer here the definition created by Robert G. Bringle, Ph.D from Kent State University for a higher education model: **"Service learning is a course-based, credit-bearing educational experience in which students: (a) participate in an organized service activity that meets identified community needs, and (b) reflect on the service activity in such a way as to gain further understanding of course content, a broader appreciation of the discipline, and an enhanced sense of personal values and civic responsibility. (Bringle & Hatcher 1995)"**

So as you see, the experts do agree on many characteristics regarding the main elements of service learning. Most would agree that the essential elements for service learning are:

- a deliberate connection between the community service and learning goals
- a reciprocal benefit to the community and the service provider
- a reflection component to demonstrate learning by service provider

The existing programs fall into four major categories: Direct, Indirect, Advocacy and Research. Direct Service entails person to person interactions, such as; teaching someone a skill. If you were to raise money for a charitable organization that would be an indirect service because it benefits the community or a group as a whole with whom you may or may not have had interactions. Advocacy is raising awareness or promoting a movement or cause and research as a form of service that takes on gathering of information and reporting information to the public. Common differences among service learning programs include whether they are imbedded in the curricula, stand alone programs, or whether the project is done individually, in small groups or by the entire class. The major philosophical discrepancies among experts arise around activity choice and evaluation. The questions that are being debated are:

- should students be part of the activity design from the impetus or can the teacher choose the activity for them?

- which forms of evaluation are most meaningful; self-evaluation, peer evaluation, teacher evaluation?

- is an evaluation tool necessary?

This is all very interesting and could be the focus of an entire book (and probably is) but I feel now that you have the necessary background needed and I want to take our discussion to describe the program I hope will be the next shift in philosophy and practice. In the next chapter, I will define and outline what I see as the difference between all these previous terms and programs and the program I have chosen to call: *"Personal Growth Initiatives"*.

Chapter Two: Introducing Personal Growth Initiatives

"The greatest gifts you can give your children are the roots of responsibility and the wings of independence."
~ Denis Waitley

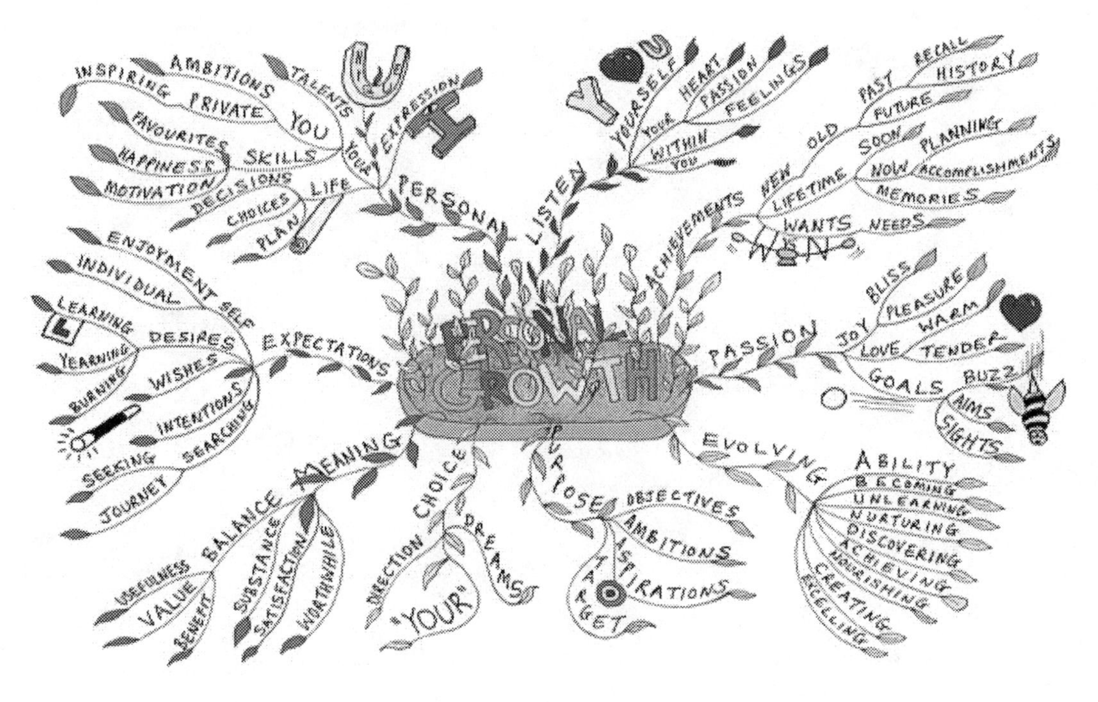

Personal Growth Initiatives are structured programs in which personal growth is the focus. The design of the experience is student driven and requires the acquisition of personal skills and knowledge.

The program defined above may sound less altruistic and community minded than the other programs. However, it is my belief that the reason many young adults are "just going through the motions" when it comes to volunteer and community service programs is because they have not developed the maturity or skill foundation to handle authentic altruism and civic responsibility. In my opinion, they are being asked to skip over many developmental steps. I believe guided personal growth experiences help them develop emotional and social maturity, in addition to skills and knowledge that can make any volunteer, community service, or service learning opportunity more meaningful.

The goal of *Personal Growth Initiative Programs is* the development of self-efficacy and personal management.

Over the years, our students have amazed us with their achievements and successes which turn out to be better than anything we could have designed for them. With the creative projects ideas that they have designed for themselves, they have taken healthy risks, gone beyond their comfort zones and faced challenges that have lead to relevant personal learning and attainment of their own personal growth goals. In most instances, the activities students choose for this project, whether intentional or not, benefit not only themselves but others as well.

None of this should be surprising if you are familiar with what Stephen Covey in his book, The Seven Habits of Highly Effective People, describes as the "maturity continuum". The maturity continuum is what he calls the natural laws of growth. All areas of growth, physical, mental and emotional have a natural growth sequence developing from dependence to independence to interdependence. In brief, as children we are dependent on others to do for us. As we mature, we become self-reliant and inner-directed and with this level of maturity and skill, we can see that doing with others is ultimately more successful and satisfying.

A well developed *Personal Growth Initiative* program will develop true leadership skills, resiliency, and produce individuals who will have a solid personal foundation. These qualities have proven to promote genuine feelings of empathy and civic responsibility.

A few years back a seventh grader who was impassioned with a quest to lessen the impact of global warming set his project goal to recruit many neighbors and family friends to sign up for a Clean Energy Option from a local utility company. He also addressed a local Kiwanis Club meeting in which he outlined the Clean Energy Option program and the downfalls of climate change and one third of those present signed up for the program. Very impressive! His project is a terrific example of a P.G.I. (Personal Growth Initiative) because it was well developed, well executed, and had him using cognitive, organizational, and social skills he had never utilized before. It also laid the foundation for even more greatness to come. This same young man, as an eighth grader, joined forces with another student and a teacher to garner more sign ups and due to the amount of resulting sign-ups they earned installation of solar panels for our school building at no cost. This young man now in high school will often contact me with information about his next event as he is determined to educate others and make the world a better place. His passion and community service have become part of who he is, not just something he did once or twice.

If you are someone who is supervising a volunteer or community service program, I strongly advocate for you to shift to a *Personal Growth Initiative* program because the participants will have greater motivation, achievements and the experience will have a longer lasting personal impact. The additional benefits promise to be astounding! Even if I were to convince you to make simple changes in an existing or future service learning programs to include personal growth goals and accountability I have no doubt that it would dramatically heighten the outcomes.

Innate in a *Personal Growth Initiative* framework is the ability to modify to meet educational needs of programs and participants. For example, the personal growth initiative program we utilize fulfills our town's health curriculum goals regarding self-esteem, critical thinking, goal-setting, self-advocacy, decision making, problem-solving, communication skills, and leadership. Another wonderful component of any P.G.I. framework is that it will lend itself to differentiated instruction so readily because it is so personalized. I will offer suggestions and give examples of modifications our students have made to suit their abilities and circumstances.

It is for these reasons, along with conviction that today's youth need more programs addressing self-efficacy and personal management that I consider it my charge to educate teachers and administrators to the value of *Personal Growth Initiatives.* I intend to reveal the ease of initiating and sustaining such a program. I will explain how to get such a program started and offer classroom materials and reproducible handouts that can be used directly with your students. I believe you will find it easy to match one of the four frameworks I will outline to your current needs and participants. In Part Two of this book, I offer detailed step by step directions to implement the program we use at F.W.M.S. and reproducible materials so you can get started right away. In Part Three, I offer descriptions and materials for alternative approaches with different focuses and assessments because you might find that one framework better suits your curriculum, teaching needs and style, and/or your students' needs over the others. So you are sure to find a P.G.I. framework that's right for you.

In the next chapter I will define and give details as to why self-efficacy and personal management are so important to develop in our youth today and how a well developed Personal Growth Initiative is a meaningful and effective tool to that end.

Self- Efficacy

"The world needs dreamers, and the world needs doers.
But above all, the world needs dreamers who do. "
~ Sarah Ban Breathnach

Self- Efficacy is a person's belief about his or her ability and capacity to accomplish a task or to deal with the challenges of life.

SELF ESTEEM +SELF-EFFICACY= SELF-CONFIDENCE

No matter the community, grade level, or subject area we teach, I feel it is safe to say that we all hope to have a positive impact on our students' self-esteem. **Self-esteem** is defined as general feelings of self-worth or self-value. Where I had been taught throughout my undergraduate and graduate coursework that self-esteem has a very strong and positive influence on academic success, some research demonstrates it may not. At best the results are inconclusive. The data does not clearly reveal which comes first, self-esteem or academic achievement. I had believed that self-esteem and academic achievement were interdependent and that a student with high self-esteem achieved better in school and that doing well in school, in turn, promoted a higher self-esteem. However, some studies I discovered also revealed instances where low self esteem was associated with higher achievement. This actually makes sense if I consider past outstanding students who were often saying things like "Am I doing this right?" and "I'm not going to be able to...". This philosophical debate has gone on for decades and probably will continue for many more. As I continued my research it did get me to thinking, if not self-esteem, then what does have an impact on success?

I have known students who may appear to have a high level of self-esteem yet lack personal qualities that could have led them to greater academic success, better decision making and life choices. What was lacking? I propose it is self-efficacy. In this day of "helicopter parenting" and school environments that foster conformity and dependency, I find that today's youth are far less genuinely confident and resilient than say when I was growing up. It is common for our youth to be told what to do step by step rather than being left to figure it out on their owns. And many young people today have been bolstered up by their parents, teachers and coaches too frequently and possibly when not excelling were told "how good they are at ..." ,"super job..." and "you're the greatest". These actions on the parts of parents and teachers were intended to raise the child's self-esteem but they may have missed the mark by not addressing the child's feeling of competence. Children usually know when they are achieving or excelling and when they are not. So, these children may <u>feel</u> good about themselves because of the external feedback they have received but lack self-confidence and self-efficacy. I do not recall where I heard this truism, but I believe it to be valid: "success is glue; it is stronger than positive reinforcement".

In my elementary school years, I enjoyed school and received very positive feedback from my teachers and peers. I was viewed as likable and cooperative. I was confident and happy about myself and with little effort did average to above average in my academics and did very well athletically. My sixth grade teacher through his unique style and lessons, taught me to challenge myself. Until that point, I had never been asked to take risks, push myself, or see myself as part of the learning process. What he taught was called back in the seventies "Humanities" which covered learning about oneself and our relationship with others and the world. One such unit incorporated lessons in history, social studies, art, math and physical education. We, students had to organize a trip to a local historical cemetery. We needed to map a route to get their on our bicycles. We had to determine how many miles we would travel and realistically how long it would take us to bike there. On the day of our trip, we had to pack and carry materials that we needed to do a tombstone "rubbing" (using charcoal you transfer the details on the tombstone onto paper). Upon our return to school using the information from our rubbings we discussed what might the lives of those people could have been like at the various times in our town's past. Through active lessons and reflections, such as the one I described, he made all the content areas meaningful to me and me an active participant. Consequently, I felt smarter and more powerful. I believe this foundation allowed me to make what could have been a difficult transition at the end of the school year. My family moved, which for me, meant starting junior high school at a new school. It was not easy at times, but I attribute my resiliency to a strong sense of self-efficacy, self-awareness, competence in working with others and a desire to learn that was fostered and practiced during the year before. I believe that this teacher and the experiences he offered not only helped me make that transition easier but laid the foundation for future achievements in and out of the school setting.

Therefore, I believe as parents and educators, we need to target the development of self-efficacy where students model behaviors such as:

- showing optimism
- being goal-oriented
- demonstrating willingness to take on challenges
- being unthreatened by change
- showing interest in learning
- displaying respect for others
- cultivating the ability to work cooperatively
- taking pride in accomplishments

Self-efficacy ultimately enhances self-esteem and leads toward self-confidence. **Self-confidence** refers to belief in one's personal worth and likelihood of succeeding that comes from a combination of self-esteem and self-efficacy.

One of my seventh grade student's P.G.I. was sparked by his realization that he had so many books that took up his book shelf from elementary school years that held no interest for him anymore and that probably so did many other kids his age. He researched and found a neighboring less affluent town that would welcome the donation of used books, so he collected slightly used elementary age appropriate books from his friends and classmates. As he prepared to call and arrange a time to bring the boxes filled with books to the school, he was filled with pride and fulfillment because he met his goal and accomplished many tasks he had never attempted before. You can see how this young man's confidence and self-worth must have been enhanced through this experience of his own making. But the best was yet to come. The principal of the school suggested that when he dropped off the books that he should stay, read one of his favorite stories to one of the classes and get to see the students who will benefit from his gift. The next day in school, he told me of the principal's suggestion which I thought was a wonderful idea but obviously had him troubled. He explained that he would love to meet the students but he was a poor reader and had often been made fun of in his early years. I let him know the principal's suggestion was simply that, a suggestion, and he could say "thank you anyway but I'll just drop the books off in the main office instead". However, I also suggested that this may be a wonderful opportunity to practice reading aloud to a receptive audience and that he could practice tonight so he would feel more confident in front of a group. I was pleasantly surprised when he told me that not only did he read a book to the elementary class but he read two. He was more proud of that aspect of his project than all of his other accomplishments. His fear, his choice, his success… true efficacy!

Using P.G.I. programs, we can give students the opportunity to go beyond their comfort zones, take healthy risks and deal with results within a framework. These experiences will teach them to assess which behaviors worked out to be strengths and which ones may need to be altered for the next time to gain what it was they had wanted to achieve all in a setting without fear, worry or anxiety. In order to master self-efficacy, I believe our students need to feel in control and powerful not because these are good qualities to aspire to have or because we tell them they have these qualities, but as result of having real life experiences that have bolstered those genuine feelings in them.

Personal Management

" A goal without a plan is just a wish."
~Antoine de Saint Exupery

Personal Management involves both a person's thinking and doing processes. The "thinking" processes include goal setting and planning and the "doing" phases include action and interpretation of the results.

THINKING + DOING= PERSONAL MANAGEMENT

We all hear on news programs and see it first hand in our classrooms that today's youth is all about "instant gratification" and almost anything they want it is just a click away. Our students tend to be impulsive, spontaneous and short term minded. Where these traits are innate qualities of youth, the access that today's children have to fast and powerful technologies have amplified them. Most have these technologies at their disposals and are ready for the next best things. Believe it or not, these technologies can also be considered factors for the growth on the maturity continuum. These afford them some measures of independence. The ability to carry cell phones has encouraged parents to give freedoms to younger age children that had not been afforded to older children in the recent past. Also, the ability to gain information and exposure to visuals on the internet has expanded the ideology of today's youth about their independence. These ideas are not all realistic or healthy but it is only fair to acknowledge that it is a reality. In order to attain the level of intellectual and emotional independence to make the most of these technological advances and to succeed in life, they need to be given the opportunity to understand and practice some fundamental management skills.

In so many ways, no matter the age of our students, they are still in the "dependent stage" of the growth process. They are directed, nurtured and sustained by others. We need to give them age appropriate experiences to test their self reliance. If we let them remain dependent, their thinking stays trapped in cycles like "you take care of me", "you can do it" and "you didn't come through for me" or "it's all your fault". This immature thinking does not lead to the want for independence and personal accountability. It is easier to have others do for us and be responsible for the results. Many children have a yearning for independence but in others, it needs to be fostered. I believe our students can be taught how to develop as independent people and value getting what they want through their own effort. This will replace the feelings of "you can" to feelings of "I can do it", "I am responsible" and "I can choose". Independent minded students become learners who feel empowered and tend to act rather than react in and out of the school setting.

GOAL SETTING AND PLANNING

The maturity required to manage one's thinking processes comes from self-awareness. Students need to be given the opportunity to investigate their imagination, dreams, concerns, strengths, weaknesses to develop the needed vision to create goals. We all know from our lives, if goals are meaningful and well chosen it helps the motivation and planning processes. We want to get things accomplished and do not mind saying "no" to something else we wanted to do in order to advance our plan.

I suppose for most of us we derived our idea of what is an effective planning style from the modeling from the adults around us growing up. Some of us may have been lucky enough to have been surrounded by adults who were proactive, balanced and effective managers. But there are many successful procrastinators who receive praise and assets for jobs well done and model to others that stress and anxiety are good motivators. Also, there are so many adults who over schedule their days, the person who can not say "no". These adults may appear important and on top of things yet due to lack of prioritizing must deal with what is most urgent and rarely gets to plan ahead or proactively. It has been the case that these models were our only source of information because very little if any instruction time in schools has been given on "how to get what you want" and "what is the most effective way to get what you want". And the tradition continues today.

As educators we want our students to thrive in the world using the knowledge and skills we have given them, however there are so many life skills we espouse but we do not directly give them the opportunity to practice. For instance, we preach to them about "being responsible" but rarely do we afford them direct skill instruction or practice and evaluation of these skills. Ask yourself, if your students could answer questions like; how does someone become responsible? what does it look like? Is it fair that adults just expect them to be able to demonstrate that skill and use it in their lives? We can do better. We should do better.

Where do we start? We offer short and long term sequential and planned opportunities to develop independent maturity. I would ask my daughter weekly when she was in elementary school, what chores would she like to contribute this week to help the household. We would discuss her choices and I'd advice her on which ones I thought were appropriate to her age and skill level and then discuss how long and when she could accomplish them. In schools, teachers might be allowing students to choose project ideas, classroom chores, rewards and consequences for behavior. Small steps like these are on the right track, but I support the use of an age appropriate Personal Growth Initiative embedded in the curriculum or standing alone to be the right tool for the job. In a P.G.I., the students are asked to create a goal, make a plan, take action on that plan and assess the results.

The development of personal management skills begins in asking students to develop self-awareness and to create goals for themselves "the why and what" of something they want to accomplish. The first step of a P.G.I. is to create a personal goal. The goal needs to be linked to their values and concerns for it to be relevant and meaningful. What do they love to do? What is really important to them? What do they wish they could change? Next, they need to make decisions and choices to act upon their values and concerns. In this sequence making a plan is justified and makes sense, the plan is the steps they need to take to get what they want. Deciding the "what and why" before taking action is a big step toward maturity. Another important step is to clearly define your expectations for what the results will look like at the project's end. Before I realized the importance of this step I would asked students at the conclusion of a project "were you successful?" and they would often not know or think they were. It is so much more satisfying in the end to know you were successful. In order to have a definitive answer after creating your goal you need to determine expectations for the results. What will have happened, what would need to have been accomplished for you to know you have achieved your goal? This step not only gives a focus to your actions during it, but also sets standards for accountability at its conclusion.

Essential skills to successfully implementing a plan are the ability to prioritize, organize and discipline. Setting priorities is about saying "yes", "no" or "later" to tasks. Students need to be taught and given practice on how to prioritize. At home, some may have had more practice than others. When they get home from school some may have their schedule predetermined for them; homework is to be done first before anything else. Even within these constraints, these children can prioritize and determine the order and amount of time spent on each assignment. In another household, a child may come home after school and be able to determine that before starting homework he/she needs to relax, have a snack and play a bit so he/she will be better able to settle down and concentrate on doing homework. However, when it comes to short and long term planning for work projects most children have been left to figuring it out for themselves with little to no guidance.

In a P.G.I. students are asked to decide what is needed to contribute to attaining their goals and then create a hierarchy of which items are necessary and urgent. Next, a long range plan can be organized by sequencing those elements by priority. Then obviously, one works to get those things that are needed to get done immediately first and can organize how to accomplish the other items that are necessary. Students can be taught that planning and thinking ahead saves stress, time and reduces the number of urgent problems arising along the way.

IMPLEMENTATION AND ASSESSMENT

Acting on the plan requires discipline. A dictionary definition for discipline is the ability to behave and work in a controlled manner. I describe discipline to my students as being about self-control and making purposeful choices and decisions. Disciplined people are thought of as being responsible, reliable and dependable because they deliver upon what they set out to do. E.M. Gray had observed "Successful people have the habit of doing the things failures don't like to do. They don't like doing them either necessarily but their disliking is subordinated to the strength of their purpose." In other words, a disciplined person executes the required task despite an impulse or desire to do something different in a given moment. This means managing time and resources according to the need of your plan. Many of my students report that the most difficult part of their P.G.I. is resisting pleasurable escapes. However, this is lessened dramatically if their project goals are personal, fun and significant to them.

Also as every good manager knows, balance and flexibility are often necessary elements to a successful endeavor. Deviation from the initial plan and making modifications may need to be done to have a successful outcome. This too can be difficult for some participants because it is difficult without much life experience knowing when it is more valued to continue to persevere and when making modifications would lead to a successful conclusion. When students have started on a course that has been approved many will not deviate without permission for believing it's the right thing to do or fear of making a mistake. I discuss with my classes that success in a P.G.I. is about learning and much of our best learning comes from mistakes. We should expect to make them; it is our thoughts and actions after our mistakes that are critical. A plan is a sketch of what we expect is needed to achieve our goal but if unexpected things arise we may need to adjust the plan. As the supervisor, be sure you give them permission to do so.

As far as assessment goes I believe as long as there is an element of self-evaluation and feedback from an adult almost any format could be used that best suit your program's needs. The reflection can be broken down into assessing preparation. The assessment is about accountability of the doer to him/herself. It is not meant to be a measure of attaining the goal. Are you surprised? This is not a goal-setting project. This is a personal growth initiative! Thankfully, nor can it be measured as success or failure based on the resulting product or action. If there is any personal growth, the doer was a success. This growth can run the gamut from doing one thing that the person had never done before to experiencing a life altering transformation. Frankly and of course, the increased level of success and goal attainment will have an expediential impact on the doer's self-efficacy.

Therefore, a person who holds a clothes drive with hopes of donating bags and bags of slightly used clothing to a local shelter yet only ends up donating one bagful could walk away with a feeling of accomplishment. A student of mine had never taken on any endeavor like this before; she called the local homeless shelter and asked what they were in need of, put flyers in her neighbors' mailboxes, made announcements at school and put a drop off box in the main office. Yet, only very few responded to her call to help others. Should she feel like a failure? No, she wanted to do something meaningful and she did but most importantly she planned something from beginning to end by herself and had never done that before. She had never called an organization or for that matter had never talked on the phone to any adult she did not know before and she reached out to her neighbors and classmates as a doer, a leader and a capable person. Was she discouraged? Of course, but when we discussed what she had accomplished in ways of personal growth and the things she had learned that could help improve such a plan in the future she eventually gave herself credit where credit was due.

Self-evaluation is important but as with the scenario above the student due to lack of perception and experience needed feedback from an adult. That is why in our P.G.I. our students must have a supervising adult who has agreed from the activity's inception to end to observe the student and provide feedback on a written evaluation form. I find that my students are able to identify mistakes they had made because they are far more practiced in finding their faults than they are at identifying their achievements. They have difficulty giving themselves credit for their actions, but often I feel they do not know of what behaviors they should be proud. Also in regards to the assessment of the activity, they may not have enough life experience to know what part of their plans might have caused problems or which modifications could have enhanced its outcome. In the scenario above, her supervising adult was her parent and this parent had found out that the local church had just had a clothing drive the previous month. When the student was told of this fact it helped her realize why her neighbors had not responded and why it had not gone as well as she had hoped. So, if she was ever to do this again one improvement she and her supervisor came up with would be to check if there had been a drive held recently in the area. They also discussed that it might have helped if she had extended the drive for a longer period of time and/or when donations were not coming in to have extended the circle of people she was involving to include family and friends.

I hope you can see how Personal Growth Initiatives are not another "teaching gimmick" or passing trend but an authentic tool to teach and give students practice in "real" life skills like discipline, responsibility, leadership, decision making, goal setting, determination, perseverance, time management and organizational skills. I can not stress enough that the program you utilize must be designed so that the activities and personal goals are significant to the current and/or future lives of the students and involve a challenge where they are asked to do something they have never done before. You will enjoy the process and be amazed with the gains in your students' maturity and successes. My students never cease to thrill and amaze me. Using P.G.I. we can give our students the opportunity to amaze themselves… how great is that!

Part Two:

What Started It All

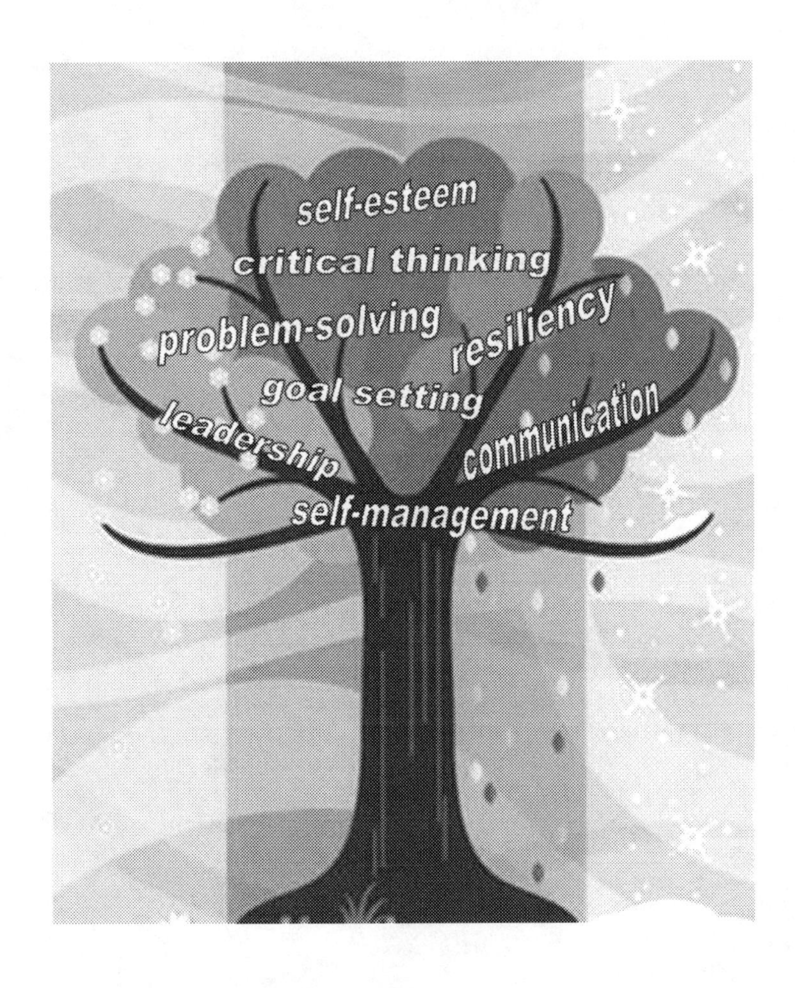

Chapter 3: Background and Description

My colleague, Cathy Hamill, created this project idea before I began teaching at Fairfield Woods Middle School in Fairfield, Ct. Excited after reading the book by Stephen Covey titled The 7 Habits of Highly Effective People she saw a link in his teachings to the seventh grade Heath curriculum. Cathy wanted to expose her health students to these concepts in a meaningful way. Her first time out she had them choose one of three suggested activities and afterward reflect upon how well they had practiced using each of the 7 habits. That was eleven years ago and the project has gone through many different phases and we believe each was an improvement upon the last. We estimate that over three thousand two hundred students have participated in this project since its inception. This year after my research for this book, we have changed the name of the project to ***Personal Growth Initiatives*** because that is the "what" or the "heart" of the project and "The 7 Habits of Highly Effective People" is the tool to focus and assess the personal growth. If you are unfamiliar with Stephen Covey's works, his first book The 7 Habits of Highly Effective People outlines philosophies and behavior changes to improve one's quality of life and one's successes. He has had many subsequent best selling books and his son even wrote one tilted The 7 Habits of Highly Effective Teens. Later in this chapter, I will review in depth each habit.

A fundamental premise of the P.G.I. at F.W.M.S. is that students take an active role in their learning. Once students learn Stephen Covey's 7 Habits of Highly Effective People they are asked to select an activity that they must initiate, organize and implement with the ultimate goal of practicing the seven habits and obtaining personal growth. Our seventh grade students' involvement in this program fulfill the health curriculum goals regarding self-esteem, critical thinking, goal-setting, self-advocacy, decision making, problem-solving, communication skills, and leadership. We feel this teaching approach offers our students to practice these essential life skills in a significant and fun way.

In this project students get to choose the activity type and activity that will be most meaningful for them. Student project ideas have included self-improvement goals, activities with friends and family, acts of kindness, and community service. Upon completion of the project, students are required to present a visual and verbal presentation to the class on how successful they were in implementing the habits.

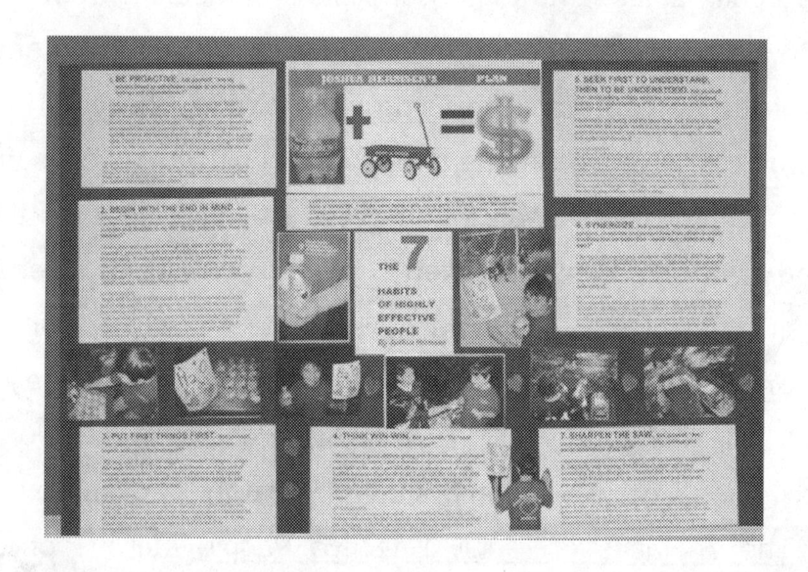

One wonderful aspect of the project's design is that the activity can be within a range from simple to complex and can be either done as a one shot deal or in a series of days or weeks. It is all up to the vision of the creator, the student. I have listed actual project ideas from former students in Chapter 7. Some have been simple but very meaningful activities that involved a special one on one connection with another person for various reasons and purposes. Often times their activity choices are in response to personal, family, community and world events. For instance, helping a family member recover from surgery or helping victims of tragic events like Huricane Katrina and the shootings at Virgina Tech. Here are a few simple but very meaningful examples; a young man helped his grandmother decorate her house for Christmas and found that since his grandfather passed away three years before she had not really decorated or celebrated the holiday and a young lady helped her brother nightly with his math homework and created fun math activities to bolster his skills. Personal connections and bonds were strengthened as these students worked on their personal management skills.Then there have been some that were complex and "over the top" based upon the visions of exceptional and dedicated participants. One young lady hosted a talent show with elementary students and charged a entrance fee with the proceeds being donated to refugees in Bosnia. She took care of reserving auditorium space, soliciting performers from the elementary school community, held tryouts, supervised rehearsals and organized an unforgetable night for what came to be the first annual talent show at that elementary school. All accomplished from the vision and labor of a seventh grade student. Amazing!

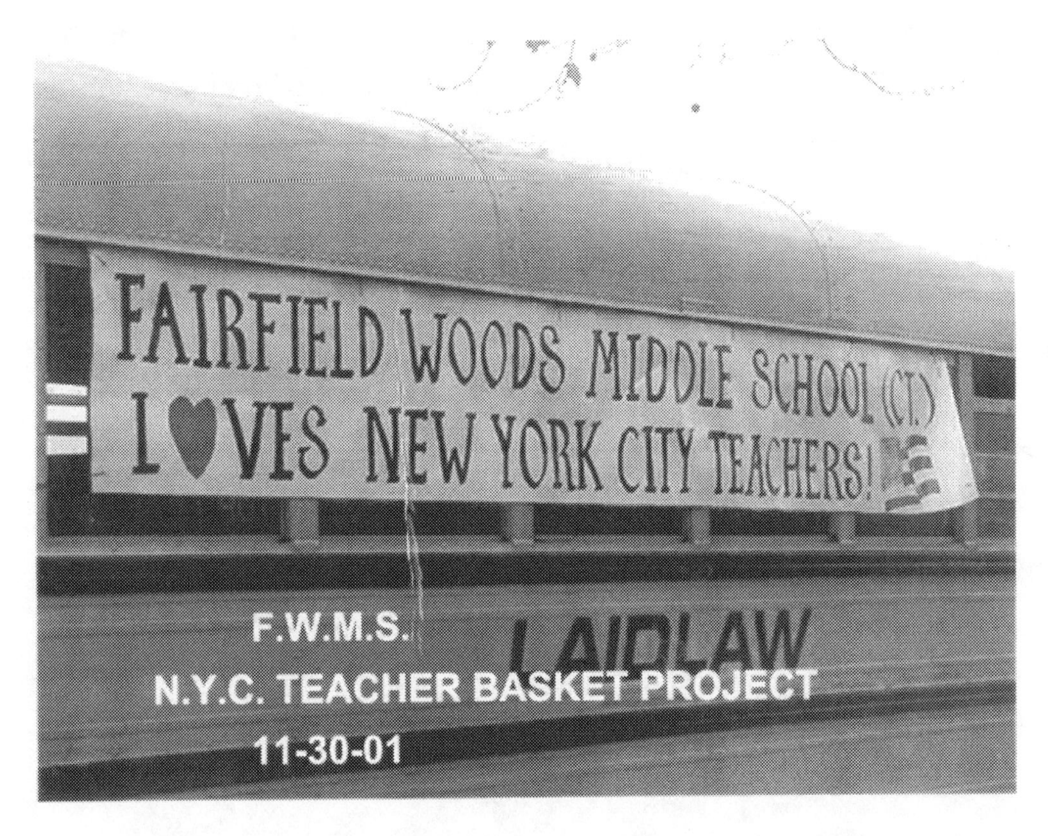

Our most publicized student project would have to have been the "Baskets for N.Y. Teacher Propject". Our town in Connecticut was shaken by the events of 9/11 by many students losing friends and family members. Many students' projects ideas were in response to wanting to help those in our community as well as in New York City. A group of four young men wanted to make a real impact and as they researched who to help they found many victim outreach programs already in place. Someone they contacted mentioned that the displaced school teachers many of whom had helped evacuate their charges to safety and stayed with them until families were located on 9/11 might have been a group overlooked. These teachers were teaching in other buildings with little to no supplies and for how long their classes would be there was unclear. These young men wanted to find a way to help these deserving teachers. They involved the whole school in the end we created thirty baskets brimming over with school supplies donated from classmates, pads made in Tech Education classes, the Art classes made beautiful ceramic dove pins, the Consumer Science classes made breads and cookies and the Health classes made "stress kits" with teas and inspirational books and sayings. It was impressive and became a school wide campaign that began in the minds of four seventh grade boys. The adminstration hired us buses to transport the baskets, students, and a few teachers to deliver these baskets to twelve New York City schools that housed these displaced classes and teachers. That day is a memory I will never forget! We were met by grateful administrators and dignitaries and they gave us police escort to visit Ground Zero. I have to believe the experience was life altering for those young men also.

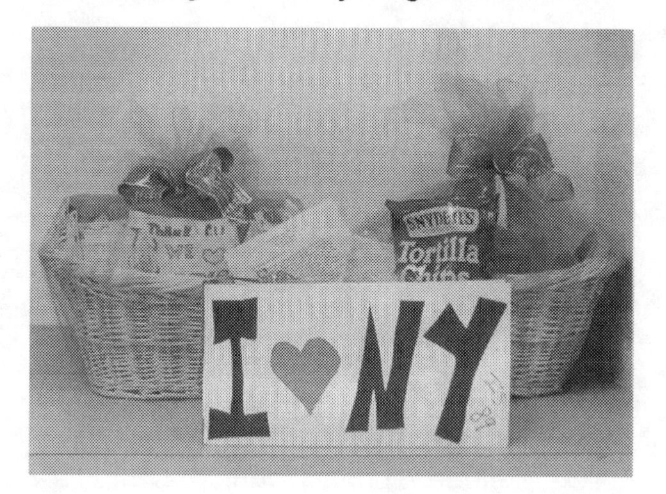

The students have enjoyed this project very much for many reasons, especially because they are given the choice of creating and designing their activity and for many it's a first time for them to take charge of an idea from start to finish. Siblings come into middle school looking forward to this project sometimes already with ideas of what they want to do. A young man graduating from high school told me recently about having found a few of the thank you notes he had received from first and second graders showing appreciation for a project he had done in seventh grade. He received between fifty and one hundred cards and still had kept some. In his email he said it made him smile knowing that he had done something nice for them and it made him feel really good about himself. He went on to say that as a young kid he got a good sense of how fortunate he was for where he lived and what he had. He learned work ethic as the whole project from beginning to end was definitely A LOT (he capitalized) of work. He got a sense of what it is like to start a project and work extremely hard at it to make it meaningful to someone else. He signed off with these remarks. "I also learned that doing things for others can not only be a good deed it can also be fun. I for one had a great time doing this project with everyone who was involved and hope the health program keeps this project for many years to come."

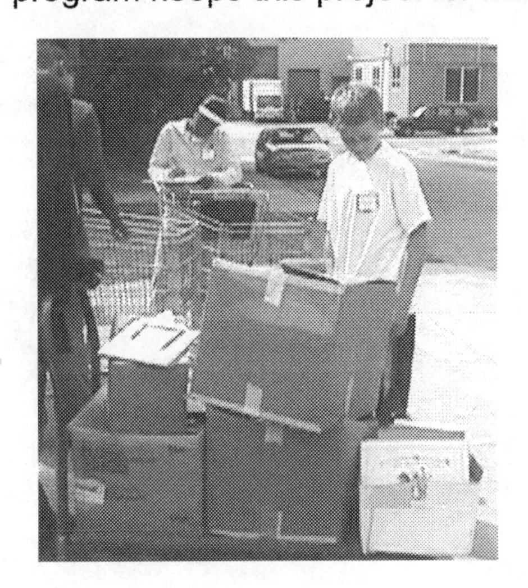

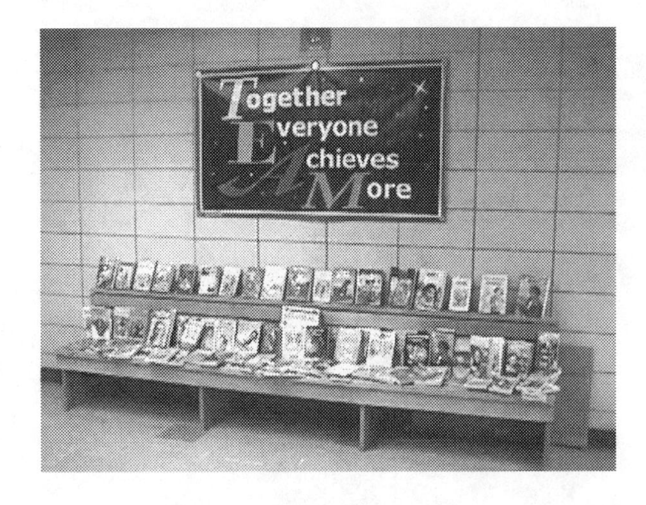

Chapter 4: Where to Begin

Steps to Implementing the P.G.I. at FWMS:

	In School	Out of School
Teaching the 7 Habits	1-2 class periods	X
Project Overview	1 class period	X
Proposal Form	(described in overview)	1 week to complete
Activity Implementation	X	Given 6-8 weeks
Teach Poster Requirements & Habits Review	1 class period	X
Student Presentations	2-4 class periods	X

TEACHING THE 7 HABITS OF HIGHLY EFFECTIVE PEOPLE

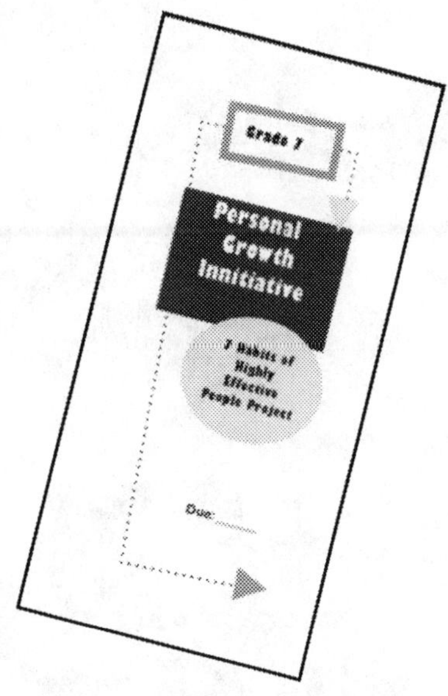

The students are given a brochure handout during our first class discussion that briefly describes the project and lists the name of each habit and a descriptive caption. This brochure is included in the Chapter 6. Students are asked to take notes during the presentation. I use a PowerPoint slide show that describes each habit's original context and then how it may apply to this project. It usually takes one forty minute period to accomplish briefly discussing all seven habits. Honestly, it may take two periods for first timers. I have included a printout of an Introductory PowerPoint slide show in Chapter 6.

On the following pages I will go into depth about each habit to give you an understanding of the habits and vocabulary to use with your students. Each section is broken down into:

- a description of Stephen Covey's habit
- my description of this habit for use with students
- a list of synonyms
- a description of how this habit carryovers into "real life"
- a list of key behaviors to practice the habit
- an explanation on how to apply this habit in a P.G.I. including examples from previous student projects and sample student write ups of how they applied the habit during their activity.

BE PROACTIVE

"There is a time to let things happen and a time
to make things happen."
~Hugh Prather

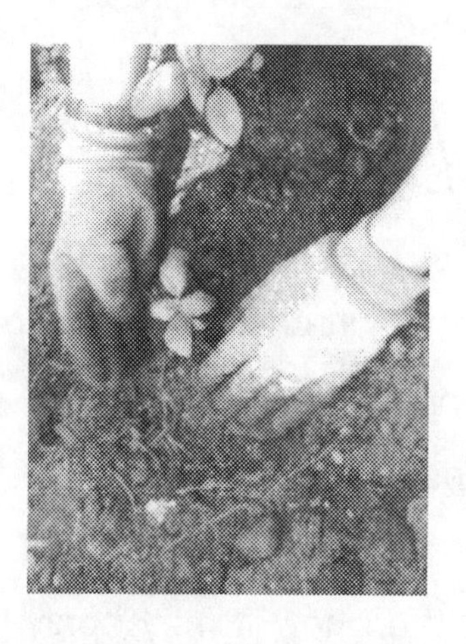

My interpretation of Stephen Covey's habit he titled *Be Proactive* is to take responsibility for your actions. The original term "proactive" was coined by Victor Frankl and it emphasized that one can either be proactive or reactive when it comes to responding to things. When you are reactive, you blame other people and circumstances for obstacles or problems. To be proactive means to take responsibility for every aspect of your life and when you do initiative and taking action will then follow. Stephen Covey argues that man is different from other animals in that he has self-consciousness. Man has the ability to detach himself and observe his own self; think about his thoughts. This self-awareness enables us to examine not only our thought processes but also our feelings and actions. Covey believes this attribute enables man to not be affected by his circumstances and due to the power of free will to choose his/her response. In a handout to my students I describe the habit in this way:

Proactive means taking initiative, not waiting for others to act first, and being responsible for what you do. The opposite of proactive is reactive. Reactive people act in response to what goes on around them (couch potatoes) and act without conviction or purpose. The actions of proactive people are deliberate and purposely based upon their principles and values.

The synonyms I use to describe proactive people are:

Innovative - Responsible - Purposeful - Visionary

When I describe this habit to my students I refer to my upbringing and how my parents would if I complained about something or commented on how I wished something could be, they always said, "well, what are you going to do about it?". In other words, they were telling me that I had the power to change or alter what was going on around me and at the very least I had the obligation to try. As young adults, my siblings and I were discouraged from complaining about situations for it was not productive to us or the world. At times I find, even now as an adult, those little voices are still in my head and I believe this philosophy has a lot to do with who I am and what I have accomplished in my life. To clarify this habit further, I go onto give examples from everyday life and ones that specifically relate to the project. One simply example I use is:

Joe is an eighth grader who lives with his single mother and two younger siblings. Lately, he finds that he is angry more often than not when he leaves for the bus each morning because his mother seems to always be on him about something. The fights are really over little things and she forgets all about them when he comes home after school. Recently it is getting so bad that his

friends and teachers are commenting on his constant bad moods. Finally, he realizes this scenario has been true since his mother has gone back to working at nights. He recognizes that she must be tired and stressed and that's why she is cranky in the mornings. So, he tells her that from now on he'll make breakfast each morning for him and his sisters so she can sleep late.

We discuss as a class why they think I would say that Joe demonstrates being proactive. They come to the fact that it is because he was not asked to help out in the mornings but when he saw the need and possible benefits of his doing so he offered to do it for the "greater good" so to speak. Joe is off to good start just by making the offer but for him to fully practice being proactive what else must he do? He, of course, must act upon his offer and consistently get up early as he said and actually do it. If he was truly practicing this habit his thought processes before making his offer to his family should have gone something like this… "I think this will be valuable for me and my family but can I really get up earlier than I do now? What can I make for breakfast? What will happen if I wake up late?" When his internal dialogue resulted in satisfactory responses then and only then should he have made the offer to his family.

This leads to a discussion on what are key personal qualities that are essential to being able to be proactive. So it makes sense that next I outline with my students **three keys to practicing this skill**, they are:

- ***To know yourself and what you feel is worthy of your energy and time***
- ***The ability to make and keep commitments and promises***
- ***To understand consequences and mistakes***

My next step in class is to assess their understanding of the habit: *Be Proactive*. I do this by trying to have them make "real life" connections to our learning so far, I ask questions like:

What words might a person use if they were Proactive, can you give an example?

Can you think of a situation when you were Proactive?

Can you think of person who often practices this habit, can you give examples of what they say or do?

Can you think of situation where someone used this habit or would have been better off if they had?

Can you think of a situation where you wish you had practiced that habit?

As I shift our discussion to how to practice this habit in our project I state that it is most important when choosing the focus of their activity. Yes it is true that this habit will be used throughout the project however to choose the most meaningful experience one must start with thinking in a proactive way. When choosing their topic I would like them to tap into their value system and to do something for which they either; see a need, have a passion for, or have always wanted to do for one reason or another. I use this thinking as a way to also incorporate the concept that Stephen Covey felt was missing when he developed his 7 Habits and that was the development of one's "unique personal significance". He has stated that his original seven habits are the road to effectiveness; it is the eight habit that is required for greatness.

I describe to my students that his eighth habit is about "passion". And no, we're not talking about the kind of passion that would really get their attention and yours. It is my belief for one to be or want to be proactive it requires a bit of what is talked about in Stephen Covey's booked titled: The 8th Habit. Therefore, with my students I do incorporate a brief discussion on this topic as well. According to

Covey, there is a great yearning, in both individuals and organizations, to discover their true "voice," to matter, to make a difference, to find greatness". The connection again that I make between this habit to our discussion of "Being Proactive" and to this project is that the most engaging and fulfilling projects are those that the students choose for themselves because of a link to something meaningful to them personally. This is at the heart of why I believe that predetermined activities in service learning programs not only diminish student motivation but also the potential gains from the experience.

To further "hit home" the concept of "being proactive" and how it can be practiced in this project I give a few examples of actual past student projects. I share about the students who love animals and choose a topic related to that passion; volunteered at veterinarian's office or animal shelter, or collected items for animals in need or rescued and one young man created a web page with pictures and descriptions of the animals at the local pound so they could find homes. Our town is primarily upper middle class and many of our students appreciate what they do have and understand that others are not so fortunate. Many of these students in wanting to help less fortunate people in neighboring towns have done so do by collecting and donating clothes, food, toys, sports equipment and books. They have also volunteered as mentors and tutors in after-school programs and community centers. Unfortunately as is true in any community, many of my students have been impacted with loved one's suffering with a diagnosis of Cancer; therefore many projects have developed out of wishes to raise awareness and money for cancer related organizations. Some students sought to create programs with activities where they saw a need or want. One young man had a passion for debating and there was no such club or activity anywhere in town so, his mission was to create a Debate Club at school and there was a young lady with a love of knitting and got a Knitting Club up and running at our school. Another repeated theme in projects has to do with the love of cooking and baking. Many students have donated the fruits of their labors or created a celebration in order to share their passion and work product. One young lady chose to share her love, knowledge and skills and teach younger students about baking. Though I have chosen many themes that are reoccurring, remember it is most important that each student feels that his/her project idea is unique and genuine to him/herself.

To wrap up the discussion on the first habit, below I have provided a write-up about "being proactive" taken directly from a student's poster. For her project she wanted to do something to comfort children staying in local hospitals because she had recently had a hospital stay. She designed, created and sold jewelry and donated the proceeds to a Hug a Bear Foundation which gives stuffed animals to children staying in the pediatric unit in local hospitals.

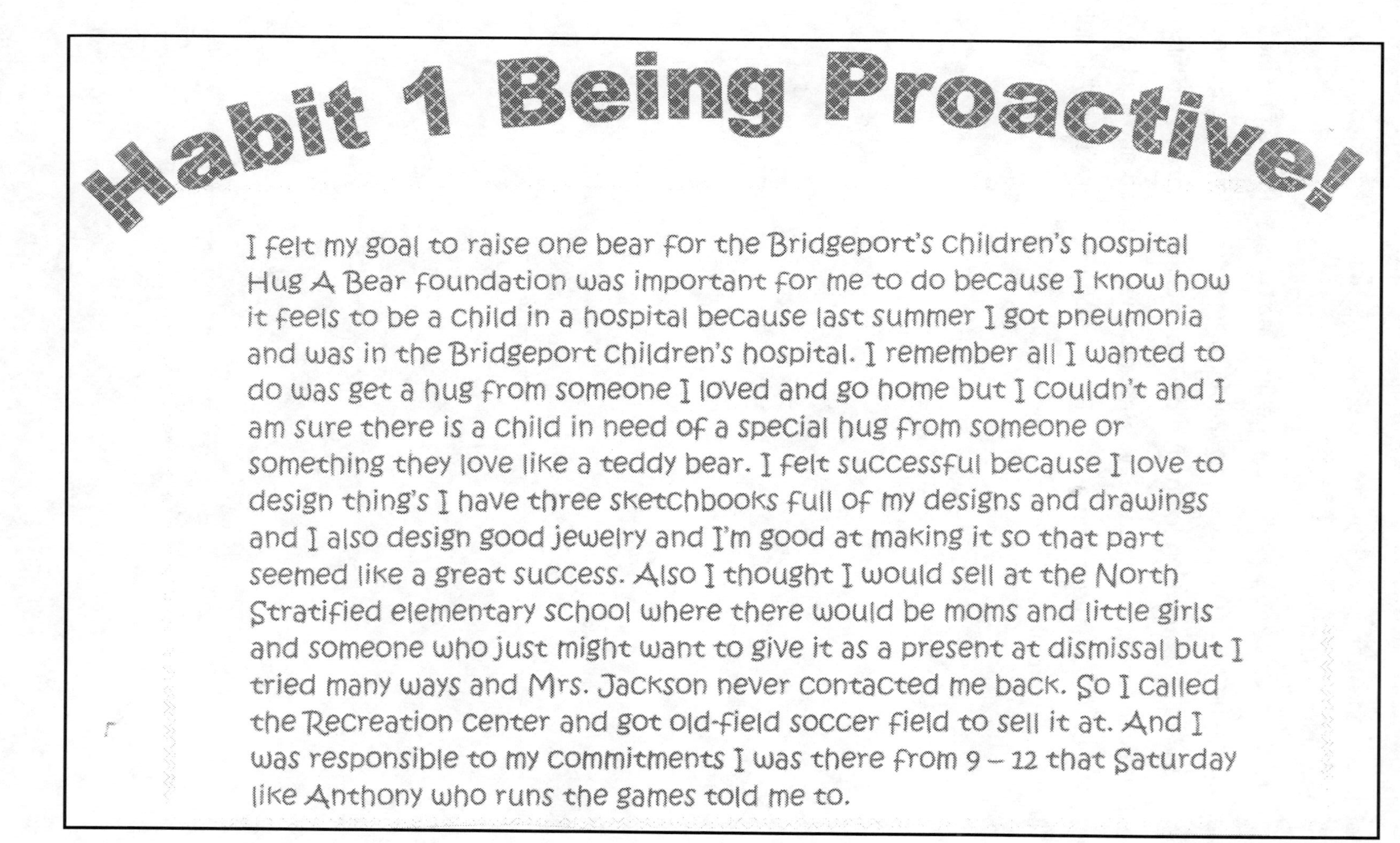

Habit 1 Being Proactive!

I felt my goal to raise one bear for the Bridgeport's children's hospital Hug A Bear foundation was important for me to do because I know how it feels to be a child in a hospital because last summer I got pneumonia and was in the Bridgeport Children's hospital. I remember all I wanted to do was get a hug from someone I loved and go home but I couldn't and I am sure there is a child in need of a special hug from someone or something they love like a teddy bear. I felt successful because I love to design thing's I have three sketchbooks full of my designs and drawings and I also design good jewelry and I'm good at making it so that part seemed like a great success. Also I thought I would sell at the North Stratified elementary school where there would be moms and little girls and someone who just might want to give it as a present at dismissal but I tried many ways and Mrs. Jackson never contacted me back. So I called the Recreation center and got old-field soccer field to sell it at. And I was responsible to my commitments I was there from 9 – 12 that Saturday like Anthony who runs the games told me to.

BEGIN WITH THE END IN MIND

" The tragedy in life doesn't lie in not reaching your goal.

The tragedy lies in having no goal to reach."

~ Benjamin Mays

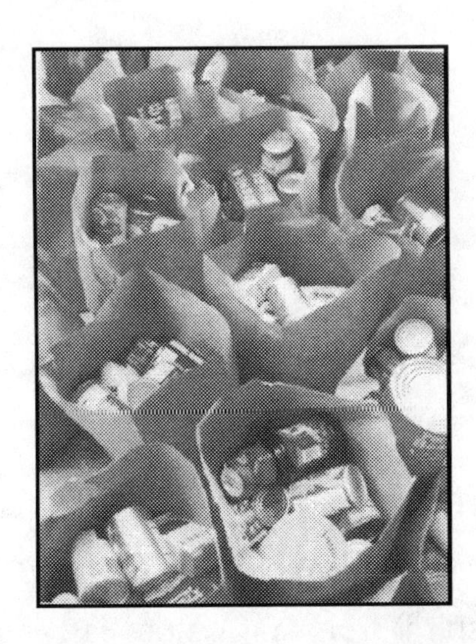

Stephen Covey's uses the habit he titled *Begin With The End in Mind* to describe what he calls "principles of personal vision". Vision as it relates to personal and work-related long term goals and he recommends formulating mission statements. These mission statements are tools to define the vision so that measurable goals can be set and focused on desired outcomes before even starting. He_espouses that these mission statements should be principle-centered and that goals should be aligned to priorities. I interpret this to mean that to be effective one should determine a goal before beginning. In order to create this goal, you must have an image of what you want to happen so it can be used as a frame of reference to measure progress. This is the mental creation piece, so to speak. One's visualization of the outcome as they would see it as gratifying. My belief is that this vision needs to also be developed based upon realistic and meaningful goals in order to lead to its fulfillment and practicing *Begin With the End in Mind* is an essential step in having that happen before the physical creation takes place.

In a handout to my students I describe the habit in this way:

Begin With The End in Mind means to begin with the image of what you want to happen so you can use it as a frame of reference to measure your progress. This is the mental preparation that needs to occur before any physical action takes place.

The synonyms I use to describe Begin With the End in Mind are:

Vision- Mission- Design- Mental Creation- Mental Preparation

When I describe this habit to my students I ask them "when your family piles into the car to go on a trip don't you always know where you are heading and what you plan to do there?" and isn't it true that before leaving someone has established where you plan to end up and what you hope to accomplish. Whether it's a shopping outing or pleasure related trip for everyone to get out of it what is hoped this needs to be determined before you leave. To clarify this habit further, I go onto give examples from everyday life and ones that specifically relate to the project. One simply example I use is:

Liz wants to have a Halloween party for her friends. She wants everyone to come to her house in costume so they can trick or treat in her neighborhood. When it starts to get late they can all go back to her house and watch a scary movie and sort their candy.

I ask the class why it is that I would say that Liz demonstrates the habit, Begin with The End in Mind. They come to the fact that it is because she has general vision of what the night will be like and would be able to measure the success of the night upon how well her image matches what in reality happened at the end of that night. Playing "devil's advocate" I might say that the night can be a total success just because she had very clear goals going into the evening and see if they agree with my contention. Eventually we establish that having a clear vision or goal does not mean the night will go as planned but because many other factors and skills are also involved to determine the ultimate outcome that night, but it's a good start. I share that the many of the habits we will be talking about deal with the issues of planning and organization that could help Liz's chances of success be greater. Yet, before we go on to discussion of the other habits I want to be certain of their understanding of this habit, *Begin With The End in Mind*, so I outline with my students what I see as three **keys to practicing this skill**, they are:

- ***To think first before you act***
- ***Visualize what you want***
- ***Determine the outcome that would please you***

My next step in class is to assess their understanding of the Habit: *Begin with The End in Mind*. I do this again by trying to have them make "real life" connections to our learning so far, I ask questions like:

What words might a person use if they were using Begin with The End in Mind, can you give an example?

Can you think of a situation when you practiced Begin with The End in Mind?

Can you think of situation where someone used this habit or would have been better off if they had?

Can you think of a situation where you wished you had practiced that habit?

As I shift our discussion toward how to practice this habit in our project I restate that it is essential to determine this vision before they start to plan their activity. I tell them that I find students when asked at the conclusion of their project "were you successful?" those who can answer "yes I accomplished what I set out to do" feel greater pride and fulfillment than students who despite having accomplished wonderful things did not practice this habit and therefore do not have a goal to asses their results. Those students seem to celebrate less their achievements and feel that their projects were somehow less important in the end. If you are vague in your goal at the start... how will you know if and when you get there?

Here is a write-up about *Begin With the End in Mind* taken directly from a student's poster. But first let me give you al little background about her project. For her project she designed a program called "Be an Allergy Pal" which she held at the local public library. She read a book called A Peanut Butter Jam to an audience of thirteen kindergarteners. Following that, she did an activity where they were asked to put foods in three categories; red (be very cautious), yellow (maybe safe) and green (generally safe). The kindergartners learned about the eight foods that commonly cause allergic reactions and discussed food allergies. Students brought home their completed craft and parents were given an informational flyer to take home.

Habit 2: Begin with the End in Mind

Before I began, I definitely had a clear vision of what I wanted to occur. I wanted four and five year old kids to learn lots about food allergies, while participating in activities and having fun. I planned to read a book called The Peanut Butter Jam, tell them the 7-8 foods that commonly caused allergy attacks, and do an arts and crafts project that would benefit them in the future. Throughout the procedure, I made sure to keep an animated and alert voice. The image I had in my mind was clearly executed, and my goal was most certainly accomplished- kids were eager to share stories and involve in conversation, and they seemed to enjoy the experience. I was very pleased with the result.

PUT FIRST THINGS FIRST

"There are no shortcuts to any place worth going"

~Beverly Sills

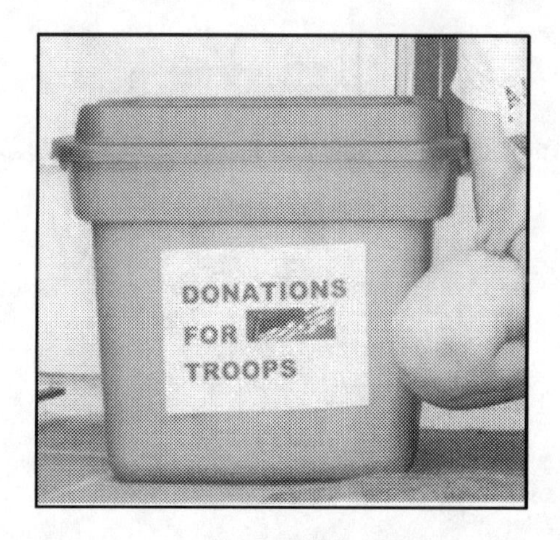

Stephen Covey's habit titled *Put First Things First* has to do with personal management. In his writings he outlines a framework for prioritizing work that is aimed at long term goals. The framework outlines how to clearly determine whether tasks are important or not and urgent or not. Therefore it is understood that an important part of time management is having a detailed work plan created in advance that focuses on benchmarks set based upon priority levels to the success of the project. My interpretation of this habit is that one aspect is about fighting procrastination and the others are about productivity and balance. It is about spending time doing what is worthwhile and making time in your life to do it. It is so much more than just planning out a project in advance, it requires that you take into account how vital is each step to the project's success and whether you can manage the needed time expenditure without sacrificing other important elements in your life.

In a handout to my students I describe the habit in this way:

To Put First Things First means to create a plan of action to achieve your personal mission and not compromise the other areas in your life. Strive to preserve a proper balance in your life by prioritizing and doing the most important things first.

The synonyms I use to the habit *Put First Things First* are:

Personal Management – Organization - Planning - Discipline

To clarify this habit further, I go give two examples one from everyday life and ones that specifically relate to the project. When I describe this habit to my students I ask them if their parents had ever told them that until your homework and chores were done there will be no watching your favorite television show. If not, imagine the situation. When you got home from school it would look something like: you would create a plan based upon the tasks needing to be done and when your show starts. You would have to take into account what tasks really need to get done to satisfy your parents, what materials you would need, time required for each task and then get it done because you really want to watch your show. To clarify this habit further, I go onto give examples from everyday life and ones that specifically relate to the project. One example that carryovers to the project is:

Kelsey wanted to help the animals at the local animal shelter. When she called she was told that she was too young to work with the care of the animals but that they are always in need of items to make the animals more comfortable when at the shelter. She decided to hold a drive to collect the items that they said that they wanted and needed. After asking her parents when they could drive her to the shelter, and checked her personal calendar, she then set a collection date and put all the details on flyers then distributed the flyer in her neighbor's mailboxes. On the collection date she visited her neighbors and loaded the bags of donation into the family car and delivered them to the animal shelter

I say to my students that Kelsey sure sounds very organized but in what ways does she demonstrates the habit, *Put First Things First*. They cite the facts that she has checked with all the other people involved in advance and did not assume she knew what to collect for the shelter but she actually found out what are the needs of the shelter. True these are important priorities that she took care of early on. Often times they mention that it sounds like she was checking tasks off a to-do list, but often they miss the fact that she considers her own availability and responsibilities which is a key element. Here is when I talk about how there are many people who take on too much, do not know how to say "no". Part of personal management is to be sure that we only take on tasks that we can do and do well. People who are unable to *Put First Things First* tend to feel stressed, overworked, and either performs tasks inadequately, late or not at all and frankly much of this is of their own making. If they had practiced putting first things first at the onset of the project, they could have devised a plan to take care of the most urgent and important things first and over the long run determine how to handle the lesser details, or in trying to plan this way they could delegate tasks to others, find the need to reestablish more realistic goals, or have found out that they should simply say "no" before committing to do the project. I also discuss that this is a learned skill and often most adults have been doing this for their children and part of maturing is to start to take on a role in these situations. I mention that they may have been mini-organizing their priorities already when deciding on how and when to do their homework. When planning their homework tasks they may choose to do the easiest assignments first, leaving only the hardest for last, or vice versa. In my opinion that is a beginning exercise for the habit *Put First Things First.* But quite frankly in our community many students admit that they are overbooked for extracurricular activities and that their parents have registered them for without their input. So not only for this project but for instant use in their lives, I outline what I see as **keys to practicing this skill**, they are:

- ***Map out steps of what needs to be done***
- ***Creating a "to do" list by priority***
- ***Keep and refer to a master schedule of commitments and responsibilities***
- ***Use a calendar or a long-term planner to track progress***

My next step in class is to assess their understanding of the Habit: *Put First Thing First.* I do this again by trying to have them make "real life" connections to our learning so far, I ask questions like:

Can you give an example of words might a person use if they were Putting First Thing First?

Can you think of celebrity, character, historic figure or person in your life that often practices this habit, can you give examples of what he/she says or does?

Can you think of a situation when you practiced Put First Thing First?

Can you think of situation where someone used this habit or would have been better off if they had?

Can you think of a situation where you wished you had practiced that habit?

As I shift our discussion toward how to practice this habit in our project I restate that it is all about planning and organizing in advance. This is a key point especially for those who are procrastinators. I try to convince them a little extra time at the start will enable them to be far more efficient and possibly make their project easier in the long run. If they determine what is most important they may figure out steps that are unnecessary and save effort right away, and when they *Put First Thing First* they often are less likely to have to go back and redo things after mistakes which reduces stress and delays. To further "hit home" the concept of *Put First Things First*, it's importance and how it can be practiced in this project I tend to start with poor examples of actual past student projects. I tell of the young lady whose goal was to throw her aunt a surprise baby shower. She had never taken on anything like this before and she was very excited. She began by asking her parents for their permission and support. Then compared her parent's schedule with her schedule and picked a date. Next she developed a guest list, wrote and mailed the invitations. She was well on her way, over the next few weeks she made decorations and researched games to play at the party. When finally, her mother asked her how she planned to get her aunt to the party unsuspecting. Oops! She had not thought of that. So, she called her uncle to see if he could become an accomplice and help to get her aunt there on time. Yet, in her conversation with her uncle she found that he and her aunt were going to be out of town the weekend that she had planned the baby shower.

My students often gasp and groan in sympathetic understanding of how everything must have fallen apart on her and see how easy such a small mistake could dismantle well laid plans. Her work almost doubled because she had to notify all the guests to reschedule, choose a new date and send new invitations. So, as a class we brainstorm what steps she should have designated as urgent and important at the onset and which could have been left for later.

Here is a write-up taken directly from a student's poster discussing how he had demonstrated *Putting First Things First.* On several occasions, this young visited a convalescent home for the elderly and performed his violin for their entertainment.

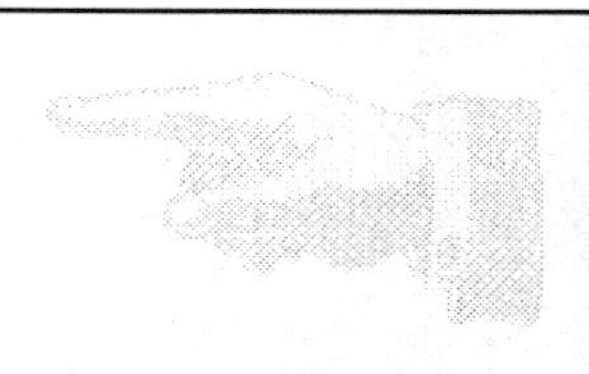

Put First Things First

Did I prioritize? Did I change my schedule and organize steps? I'll tell you what I did. And you decide. Before knowing it was a good habit, I always prioritized and used organizational skills. I just was unaware of the great benefits of implementing this habit. I skipped Karate and rescheduled my dentist appointment in an attempt to go to the Jewish Home. I had to get ready quickly in order to get to JHE on time. I first sat with my mom to discuss ideas regarding the project. Then, with the help of my mom, I found dates and times on which I could possibly play the music for the elderly at JHE. Afterwards, I contacted Ms. Shelly Berman, volunteer coordinator at JHE. Every day, I followed the instructions she, originally, gave me. Every time I went to JHE, I knew exactly what I wanted to do, as I planned it out ahead of time. As you can probably see from this description, I clearly prioritized and took good organizational steps to accomplish my project.

"A healthy attitude is contagious. Don't wait to catch it from others. Be a carrier." ~ Tom Sheppard

THINK WIN / WIN

"It is one of the beautiful compensations of this life that no one can sincerely try to help another without helping himself."
~Ralph Waldo Emerson

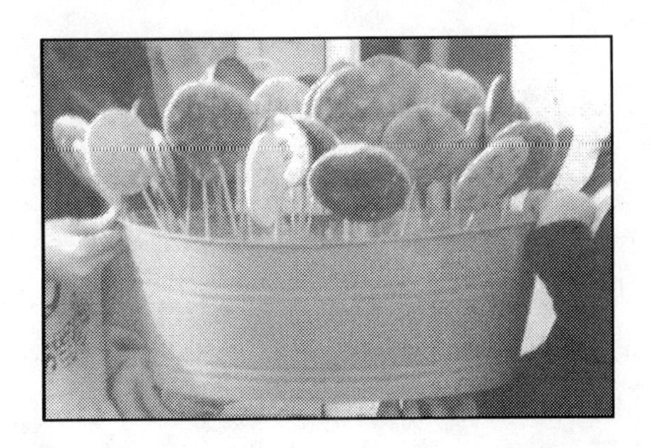

Stephen Covey's habit he titled *Think Win/Win* relates to principles of mutual benefit. He considers this habit necessary for interdependence. It is a frame of mind and heart that constantly seeks mutual benefit in all human interactions. Covey sees life as cooperative, not a competitive arena and that one person's success is not achieved at the expense or exclusion of the success of others. He describes this thinking to not to have to have it be my way or your way but that there can be a third alternative; a better way. With a Win/Win solution all parties feel good about the decision and feel committed to the action plan or in the cases where a win/win deal can not be achieved, accept that agreeing to a no deal may be the best alternative.

In a handout to my students I describe the habit in this way:

To Think Win/Win means to seek those situations, solutions, projects, and relationships that are mutually satisfying. When you come upon a problem, you are optimistic when trying to solve it and know when you walk away from it that you still learned something from it.

The synonyms I use to describe someone who demonstrates Think Win/Win are:

Respectful - Positive - Cooperative - Considerate- Flexible

When I describe this habit to my students I come at it in two ways; the *Think Win/Win* mindset and *Think Win/Win* actions that demonstrate the mindset. Firstly, I ask them if they know anyone who just seems positive all the time even when things go badly. And does that person you are thinking of seem to find a way out of the bad times faster than other people, especially those who get all negative and complain. When we agree that that is typically true, I explain that positive energy forces people forward where negative energy holds them back. Also negative thinking tends to isolate a person, where people may be drawn to help and encourage a person with a positive attitude. Next, I address the actions that create Win/Win and these include problem solving in a way that considers and respects all parties and attempts to arrive at a mutually satisfying situation. However, a problem or conflict does not have to be present to *Think Win/Win*. Any time a person acts to improve a situation for another it is demonstrating *Think Win/Win* as long as it is not at his/her expense or in any way compromising his/her own needs. To clarify this habit further, I go onto give examples from everyday life and ones that specifically relate to the project. One simply example I use is:

It is a beautiful day outside and Tom's mother asks him to clean out his closet and get rid of all his clothes that he has outgrown to make room for some new ones. Though he is not thrilled at first to do this as he is sorting his clothes he remembers someone at school is holding a clothing drive to benefit the local homeless shelter. So, he decides to bag all his unwanted clothes and donate them. He suggests that if everyone in the family does the same thing not only will they help more people it will also open up closet storage in their house.

We discuss as a class why they think I would say that Tom demonstrated *Think Win/Win*. They come to the fact that where he could have easily been bad tempered about having to do this task he chose not to go there, and by not going the way of negative thinking he turned a simple chore into a very productive and mutually beneficial task. He benefited, his family benefited, and the residents at the homeless shelter also benefited. Before we go on to discuss how this habit can be practiced in this project I want to be certain of their understanding of this habit, *Think Win/Win*, so I outline with my students what I see as three **keys to practicing this skill**, they are:

- ***Think "we, not "I"***
- ***Accept a compromise when necessary to find mutual benefit***
- ***Try to stay positive and make changes for the better***
- ***Seek to get involved with situations that hold mutual benefit***

Here as I had done with the other habits, I would next assess their understanding of the habit by asking them to make "real life" connections to our learning so far, I ask questions like:

What words might a person use if they were Thinking Win/Win, *can you give an example?*

Can you think of a situation when you practiced Think Win/Win*?*

Can you think of person who often practices this habit, can you give examples of what they say or do?

Can you think of situation where someone used this habit or would have been better off if they had?

Can you think of a situation where you wish you had practiced Think Win/Win*?*

As I shift our discussion forward to how this habit relates to our project, I state that this habit will be used throughout the course of the project and can hopefully become part of their daily lives starting now.

I share my belief that competitive personalities tend to use more energy and unifying personalities radiate energy. And that practicing this mindset and complementary behaviors can make you the type of person that people want to be around and feel good to be around. To further "hit home" the concept of *Think Win/Win* and how it can be practiced in this project I give an few example from an actual past student project. The story involves a young lady who set out to bake a cake with her younger sister for an elderly neighbor. Her intention was to do something nice for the elderly woman and she involved her sister only because her mother had said she was going to have to watch her at that time anyway. To her amazement she really enjoyed her sister's company, which she rarely took time to do much lately and found spending time with her sister was one of the things she liked best about the project.

The student write-up I have chosen as an example is from a young man's project I referred to earlier in the book. His project involved raising awareness about climate changes and getting community members to sign up for the *Clean Energy Choice Option* with the local utility company. I have chosen to share his write-up about his practice of the *Think Win-Win* habit.

Habit 4
Think Win-Win

This habit was one of my strongest throughout this project, no matter how discouraging some things could get. In past projects, this habit has cost me so I really attempted to be optimistic throughout the project. I feel this positive attitude had a benefit to the others I was working with, as I had hoped. Through the project, I looked to spread my optimism and hope for many signups. A classic example of my optimism affecting others was when we had a lack of success on the school level, and those working with me including my mom was worried. However, again and again I told her that when I went to the Kiwanis Club I would receive signups and about a third of the people there did sign up. When I felt pressured because Mrs. Cox was going away and I needed her approval for the project was a time where I needed to think that I will do fine and things will be o.k. I tried to persuade myself that just by raising awareness, I would be doing well and if I were to get signups, I would have done a good job. These are some of the ways I thought win-win in order to help my own spirits as well as the spirits of those I was working with.

SEEK FIRST TO UNDERSTAND, THEN TO BE UNDERSTOOD

"A single question can be more influential than a thousand statements."
~Bo Bennett

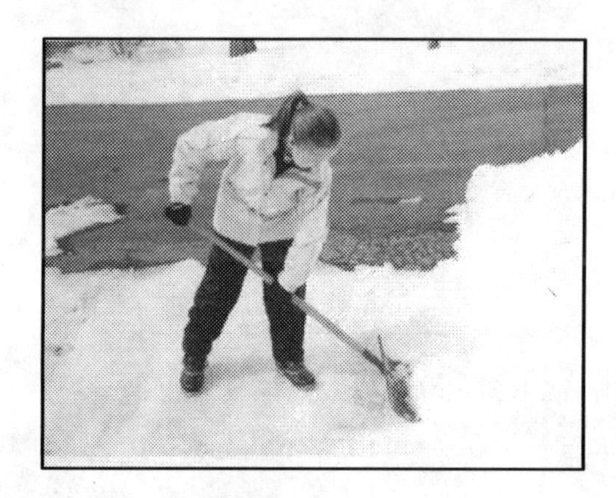

Stephen Covey to describe his concepts related to principles of mutual understanding he named the habit *Seek First to Understand, Then to Be Understood*. He teaches that the most important principle in interpersonal relations is to first seek to understand the other person, and only then to be understood and that these are critical to reaching win/win solutions. Seeking to understand takes consideration, seeking to be understood takes courage. In his book, this concept became most clear to me when he defined three sequentially arranged words from the early Greeks: ethos, pathos, and logos. Ethos is your personal credibility, the faith people have in your integrity and competency. Pathos is the empathetic side, it's the feeling. It means that you are in alignment with the emotional thrust of another person's communication. Logos is the logic, the reasoning part of the presentation. He concludes that the sequence ethos, pathos, logos- your character, your relationships and then the logic of your presentation are essential to effective communication. I describe this habit to my students in two steps, first by first defining effective listening. Effective listening is putting oneself in the perspective of the other person, listening emphatically for both feeling and meaning. It may require inquiry and discussion to be certain you have accurately understood their intention. The second piece relates to your response to what information you received through effective listening. Next, I explain that it is best for one to not only use that information in creating one's response and if you demonstrate that it is being done purposefully the recipient of your advice or the person you wish to work with will no doubt be more receptive to what you have to say. Another advantage to this approach is that the initial response will have already made steps to bringing both parties' expectations closer to one another. One's response needs to be clear, demonstrate logic, as well as the feeling and meaning behind the words for effective communication to have taken place.

In a handout to my students I describe the habit in this way:

> ***Seek First to Understand, Then to Be Understood means to listen with genuine interest to fully understand both the feeling and meaning of the other person's words. Effective communication is taking into account the perspective of that person in creating your response and then clearly sharing your thoughts and/or expectations.***

The synonyms I use to describe a person who Seeks First to Understand, Then to Be Understood are:

Perceptive- Empathetic- Articulate- Good Communicator

When I describe this habit to my students I ask them if they had ever been in a situation where another person is trying to convince them of their point of view while not even considering yours. "I've done this a million times, come on... I know you are going to love it". Or had they ever been in the situation when they were sharing a story or feelings and the receiver starts giving their opinions and advice when you had not even asked for any. Of course, we have all been in these situations because generally speaking people are not great listeners. Most people have not been taught or seen modeling of *Seek First to Understand, Then to Be Understood.* And in most of the current media whether it be print or visual, people are encouraged to share their opinions over that of others and to demonstrate their wisdom by telling others what they should do. These techniques while they grab ratings do not tend to lead to greater understanding and progress. To clarify this habit further, I go onto give examples from everyday life and ones that specifically relate to the project. One simply example I use is:

Sam is riding home on the "late" school bus because he missed his regular bus. What a bad day he had had, if anything could go wrong it did but instead of dwelling on the bad he shifts his thinking to the chocolate chip cookies that his mother made this morning and how great it will be to have a tall glass of milk and some of those cookies. As he gets off the bus, he remembers his little brother will have gotten home ahead of him because of the bus fiasco and thinks he better not have had those cookies. He is fuming when he sees the empty cookie plate and his brother watching TV in the kitchen. *(I usually have the kids tell me what they think happens next- and they usually concur that some sort of violence is about to happen)* ***Sam pushes his little brother off the couch as he yells, "I can't believe you ate all the cookies!" As the brother continues to deny it, Sam does not listen and gets louder and madder, more and more aggressive only stopping due to the until ringing phone. It's their mother and the little brother tattles on Sam and he gets grounded for two days. Then the little brother relays the reason for her call is because she forgot to leave a note saying that she left a few cookies for them in the cookie jar because she took most of the cookies to work for a coworker's birthday party.***

I ask the class why they think I chose this story to talk about *Seek First to Understand, Then to Be Understood*. They come to a consensus that it is because Sam did not practice this habit and the situation could have worked out so much better if he had. I ask them to rewind the story and to create a new ending which involves Sam practicing the habit. Often their versions include Sam asking his little brother in a calm voice "where are the cookies?" and when he says "huh?, I don't know" he follows up with "do you know what happened to them?" and again the brother says "no". With some prompting, they have Sam go on to tell his little brother of his very bad day and how he was so looking forward to those cookies. No fight occurs, no grounding but often sometimes the story leads to them brainstorming and looking for another treat or baking a new batch of cookies for themselves. In order to be certain of their understanding of this habit, *Seek First to Understand, Then to Be Understood,* I outline what I see as three **keys to practicing this skill**, they are:

- ***Ask questions to clarify that you understand correctly***
- ***Probe for further meaning by nonverbal cues (body language)***
- ***Present your ideas and needs clearly, and specify how they relate to the listener***

My next step in class is to assess their understanding of the Habit: *Seek First to Understand, Then to Be Understood.* I ask them to make "real life" connections to our learning so far, I ask questions like:

What words might a person use if they were Seeking First to Understand, Then to Be Understood, can you give an example?

Can you think of a situation when <u>you</u> practiced the habit Seek First to Understand, Then to Be Understood?

Can you think of situation where someone used this habit or would have been better off if they had?

Can you think of a situation where you wished you had practiced that habit?

As I shift our discussion toward how to practice *Seek First to Understand, Then to Be Understood* during this project I usually use examples again of those students who learned from not practicing this skill well. One young man's project proposal stated that he would do chores for his grandmother who just had a hip replaced a few Saturdays in a row. Great idea and his planning was good and when he got there he told her that he would have time to do the dishes, dust, vacuum and pick up sticks in the yard before his parents would be back for him. He did just as he explained and did a good job but was somewhat disappointed with his grandmother's lack of enthusiasm. Later he overheard a conversation between his mother and grandmother where his grandmother said she appreciated his help but that even in her condition she can and does enjoy doing the dishes and dusting, but would rather he did the laundry next week because she can not go down the stairs to the basement. Where this young man did a very good job executing the tasks he had outlined, he missed the first step which was to ask her what her expectations were for this situation.

I explain to my students that this tends to be the most common area that mistakes are made because many have had little experience and practice. To this point in their lives, often they have been told what to do. Therefore in this project when they are determining the "what" they are going to do they often make errors that effective communication could have prevented. Another such example involves a young lady who did a wonderful job planning and implementing an activity with a second grade class. After the teacher praised her on how well she had done he said "see you next week". The problem here was she had not clearly articulated to the teacher that her expectation was for this to be a one time experience. So instead of feeling proud and accomplished, she left feeling embarrassed and uncertain about what to do next.

Here is a write-up taken directly from a student's poster discussing how he demonstrated *Seek First to Understand, then to Be Understood*. His project was to design a web page for his father's friend's business.

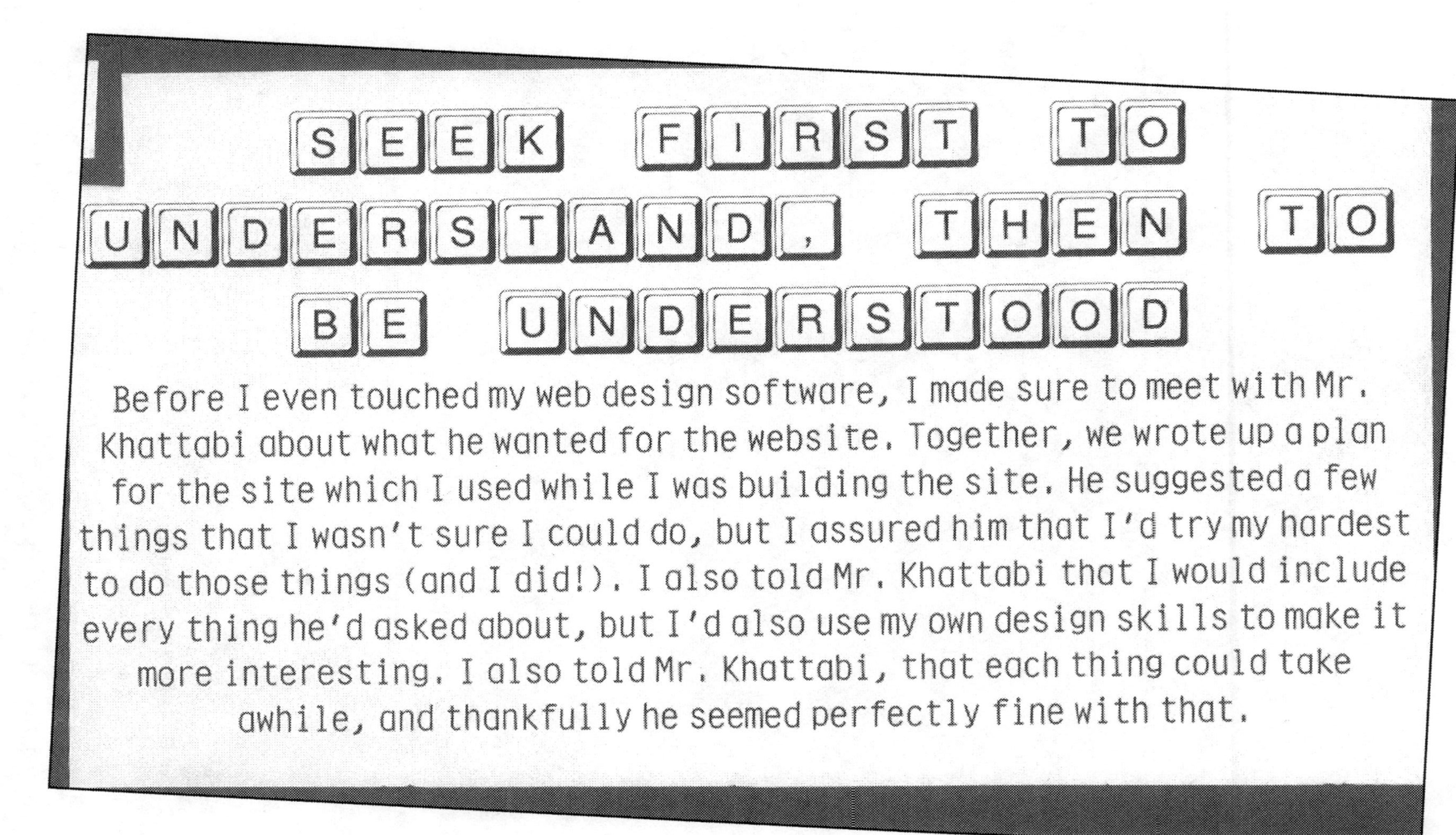
SEEK FIRST TO
UNDERSTAND, THEN TO
BE UNDERSTOOD
Before I even touched my web design software, I made sure to meet with Mr. Khattabi about what he wanted for the website. Together, we wrote up a plan for the site which I used while I was building the site. He suggested a few things that I wasn't sure I could do, but I assured him that I'd try my hardest to do those things (and I did!). I also told Mr. Khattabi that I would include every thing he'd asked about, but I'd also use my own design skills to make it more interesting. I also told Mr. Khattabi, that each thing could take awhile, and thankfully he seemed perfectly fine with that.

SYNERGIZE

" As we grow as unique persons, we learn to respect the uniqueness of others"
~Robert H. Schuller

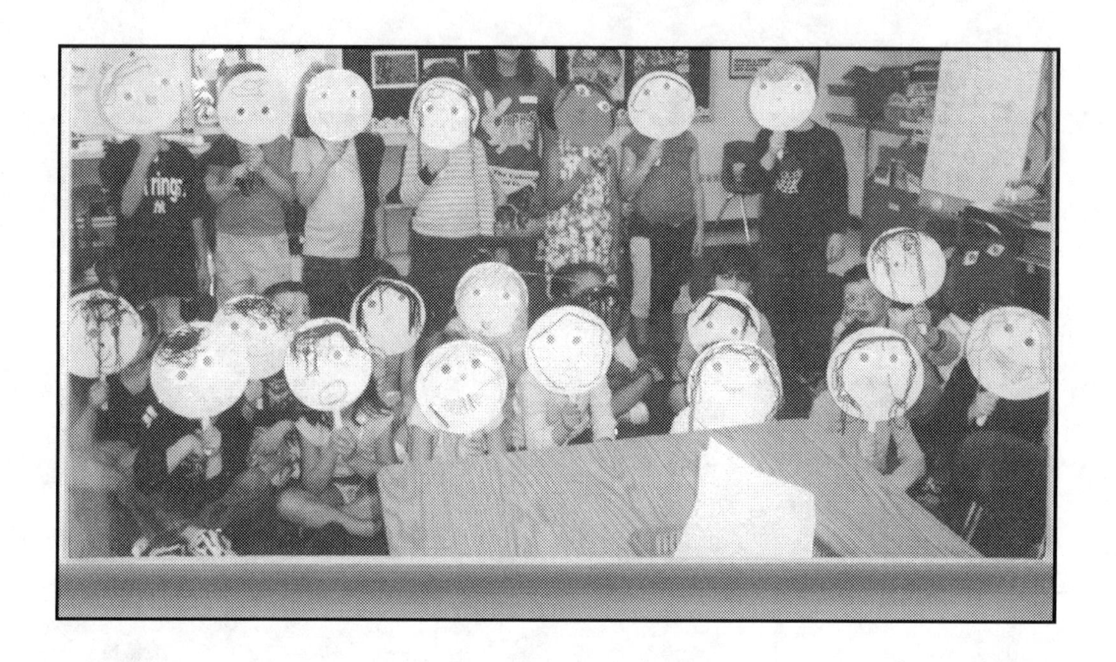

Stephen Covey's uses the term Synergize to explain the habit that he calls "principles of creative cooperation". I have heard it referred to as "creative collaboration" and I think the term collaboration as compared to cooperation gets more to the heart of the habit's true meaning. *Synergize* describes the creative process that produces a whole that is greater than the sum of its parts. According to Covey, the essence of synergy is to value differences- to respect them, to build on strengths, to compensate for weaknesses. Through mutual trust and understanding and practicing the other habits, most especially *Think Win/Win* and *Seek First to Understand, Then to be Understood*, people can go the next step to create new alternatives- something that was not there before. Synergy catalyzes, unifies and unleashes the greatest powers within people. Covey explains the process to be when parties act together on one side, even though their beginning viewpoints might be at odds, they look at the problem, try to understand the needs involved and work to create a third alternative that will meet them. Using his terms it gets beyond, "my way" versus "your way" to "the high way" which is the best solution created from new options and ideas. I make the distinction between a compromised and synergized solution as where both are mutually beneficial it is only in a solution produced from synergy that the product is better than what either of them originally proposed.

In a handout to my students I describe *Synergize* in this way:

> ***Synergize means to work with others, cooperate, and be open to new ideas or ways. Through mutual trust and understanding problems can be solved and ideas created that are obtained through a joining of individual ideas and strengths.***

The synonyms I use to describe a person who practices Synergize are:

Open Minded- Cooperative- Collaborative- Alternative Seeking

When I describe *Synergize* to my students I ask them to think if there had ever been a time when they were getting together with their friends and everyone wanted to do something different. Maybe it became more like a negotiation where some friends were not going to back down from their ideas and others did not really care too much and just wanted it to get settled and it seemed like it was never going to get resolved. But instead of a huge disagreement, deciding to do nothing at all, or breaking off into small groups and doing different things, someone in the group came up with a suggestion that was different from all the rest that everyone got excited about it and together you all decided that it was an even better idea. Well, if you have a similar memory than it could be said that you and your friends have begun practicing synergy. I then ask them to think of a person they know who is known to say something like "It's my way or the highway!" and are unyielding to listen to different people's points of views. I do not encourage them to share any names but ask them whether they like to work with that person and why or why not? I explain that everyone likes to feel that their interests, thoughts and feelings have relevance (this goes back to *Seek First to Understand, Then to be Understood*) but more importantly regarding synergy it is about honoring one another's differences to gain perspective and skills not already considered. The "it's my way or the highway" type thinker minimizes the potential for personal grow and dramatically limits his/her effectiveness and success potential. It takes courage and maturity to synergize. In order to gain new insights and options you have to be able to share honestly your thoughts, to be open for criticism, and then also consider another's needs and ideas. To clarify this habit further, I go on to give examples from everyday life and ones that specifically relate to the project. One simply example I use is:

Brian had collected a lot of books that he planned to donate to an elementary school in a less fortunate area of town that does not have classroom libraries. When he calls the principal to get the details about where and when he should drop off the books, the principal suggests that he give the books directly to children in a classroom. Brian explains that he feels he would be embarrassed doing that because it would look like he was doing this to get praise from the children and that was not what he was after. So, the principal explains that he would like his students to meet him because it will bring home the fact that "everyday" young people can make positive differences in this world. The principal suggests that when he drops off the books to the school that he stays and should read one of his favorite books to one of the classes. He did just that. After he read the book to the class the children did thank him but they quickly shifted to asking him about the other books as they began investigating the books he had brought. It was an amazing experience, not at all awkward, and better than he ever imagined.

I ask the class why it is that they that I would say that Brain demonstrates the habit, *Synergize*. They see pretty clearly that because Brian was open to the principal's suggestions the resulting situation was something he would not have come up with himself, the solution satisfied his and the principal needs, and turned out to be more gratifying than the original plan would have been.

Though this habit in theory is pretty easy to understand, it is one that many of my students will have had little practice and may not know where to start so to further their understanding of *Synergize*, I outline what I see as three **keys to practicing this skill**, they are:

- ***Ask about prior knowledge or experience from others***
- ***Share your thinking and plans and invite suggestions***
- ***Seek new alternative and brainstorm with others***

My next step in class is to assess their understanding of the Synergize. I do this again by trying to have them make "real life" connections to our learning so far, I ask questions like:

What words might a person use if they were Synergizing, can you give an example?

Can you think of celebrity, character, historic figure or person in your life that often practices this habit, can you give examples of what he/she says or does?

Can you think of a situation when <u>you</u> practiced the habit Synergize?

Can you think of situation where someone used this habit or would have been better off if they had?

Can you think of a situation where you wished you had practiced that habit?

As I shift our discussion toward how to practice this habit in our project I emphasize that this is their project based upon their vision and plan. Where I want them to be open to ideas and suggestions they ultimately have the "veto power". I give them permission to listen respectfully to adults' suggestions, most especially their parents, and say "thank you and I appreciate your opinions" but they do not have to follow their advice. One such example was when a young man who loves science chose to visit his former fourth grade teacher's current class to do an experiment on electricity. He researched and found what he thought was an exciting activity to do with the class. A few days in advance, he brought all his materials to demonstrate his planned experiment to the teacher for his opinions. The experiment went as expected and he was very pleased. The teacher agreed that it went well but he chose to show him the experiment that he usually uses to demonstrate the same concepts in case he wanted to do that one instead. After seeing the teacher's experiment, the young man thanked him for showing the alternative to him but said that he still would like to use the experiment that he had originally planned and he did. The students, the teacher and the young man enjoyed the experience and the experiment worked as hoped.

I explain to my students that sometimes when we listen to different viewpoints, the process itself can take us down different paths; it could bring us to where we think the suggestions are worthy of further investigation, or it can cement in our minds the value of our previous ideas, or it could help us come up with another way altogether. However, I caution students that this is a difficult habit and one for which they usually have little experience. Where this young man had a clear vision of how he wanted his project to unfold in order to satisfy his mission. Sometimes others are less inclined to alter plans for other reasons. They may have practiced Begin With the End in Mind and had a predetermined goal, however they lack experience and confidence to deviate from that plan because they lack the judgment to determine whether their mission could be better served by modifying that course. Or I have found that what holds back some young adults is that they are not clear enough about their own needs and ideas to know if someone else's proposals do or do not support them. However, I also caution students that sometimes people of all ages are intimidated into using other peoples' suggestions due to a want to appease them and that, of course, is not true synergy.

To conclude discussion of this habit, I try to bring home the importance of practicing this habit not only in this project, but at home, with their friends as well as in small group work in other classes because to master this habit is especially important to their relationships and work successes now through adulthood. To see personal differences as gifts rather than obstacles will open you to meaningful, trusting relationships and it can lead to the development of the mindset of a "life long learner" who is always growing and consistently looking for the new thing, the new way, or the new idea.

To wrap up the discussion on this habit, I offer a write-up about Synergize taken directly from the same student's poster. As in the last habit, he was the young man who designed a web page for his father's friend's business.

SYNERGIZE

I worked with Mr. Khattabi a lot on his website. When he came to check the website, there were some places where he found mistakes or something he wanted added. I listened to him and his advice on what I should do for his website, and I fixed all the mistakes while he was there. For the things he wanted added, it would take a little too much of his time to do it while he was over, so I simply told him I'd do it when he left – and I did. I'm glad he helped me because I might have had some mistakes without his help and commentary.

SHARPEN THE SAW

"Today you are You, that is truer than true, There is no one alive who is Youer than You."
~Dr.Seuss

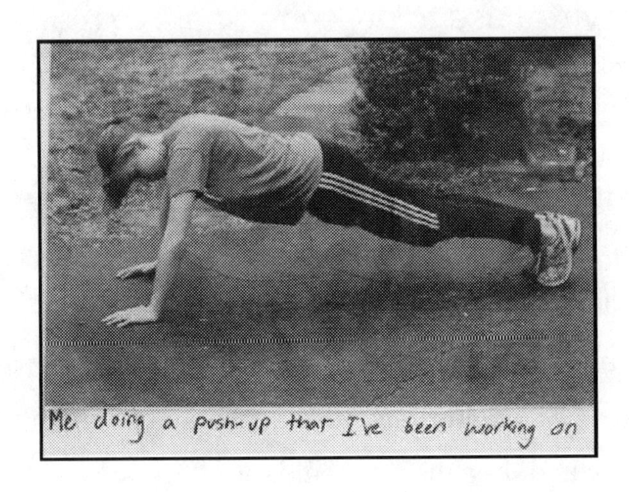
Me doing a push-up that I've been working on

My interpretation of Stephen Covey's habit he titled *Sharpen the Saw* focuses on balanced self-renewal, regaining what he calls "production capability" by engaging in carefully selected recreational activities. Covey also emphasizes the need to sharpen the mind. Under these principles of balanced self-renewal he feels it is essential to take time out from production to build production capacity through personal renewal of the physical, mental, social/emotional, and spiritual dimensions an to maintain a balance among these dimensions. A simply analogy favored by Stephen Covey is that you are the saw; and so Sharpening the Saw is about improving yourself. To internalize this habit, you must ask yourself the following questions: what am I doing to keep physically healthy, to sharpen my mind, to feed my personal needs, and to align my vision and personal mission with the universal greater values of mankind?

In a handout to my students I describe the habit in this way:

Sharpen the Saw means to take time to reflect and rejuvenate. This sharpening allows for personal growth and change. It promotes continuous balancing of one's mental, physical and spiritual health.

The synonyms I use to describe *Sharpen the Saw* are:

Self Renewal- Replenish- Recharge- Personal Growth

When I describe this habit to my students, I refer back to "the twelve ingredients of health" which is the definition of wellness upon which we base our curriculum. We teach to attain wellness one must maintain and balance the three areas of health; physical, mental and spiritual. This can be done when attention is given to satisfying the four daily requirements of each area of health. Therefore, the term "the twelve ingredients of health" represents the three areas of health multiplied by the four daily requirements to equal the twelve ingredients of health. Here are the definitions for the three areas of health and the four daily requirements.

PHYSICAL HEALTH: any biological function related to the systems of the body

MENTAL HEALTH: gaining of knowledge and the ability to reason ... for example: to learn, make decisions, evaluate, calculate, identify, etc.

SPIRITUAL HEALTH: how you feel about yourself and interact with the world around you using the greater values of mankind.

THE FOUR DAILY REQUIREMENTS:

FOOD= fuel and nutrients to energize

REST = allowing the health area to be still, taking a break

EXERCISE = work output, performing tasks

ELIMINATION = exiting of waste

THE 12 INGREDIENTS OF HEALTH

		High Quality Behaviors	Low Quality Behaviors
PHYSICAL HEALTH			
	FOOD:	apple	candy
	REST:	restful sleep	disturbed sleep
	EXERCISE:	swimming	bowling
	ELIMINATION:	exhaling CO_2	dry cough
MENTAL HEALTH			
	FOOD:	academic information	cartoons
	REST:	vacation	drug abuse
	EXERCISE:	reading	doodling
	ELIMINATION:	correcting mistakes	forgetting information
SPIRITUAL HEALTH			
	FOOD:	love	false pride
	REST:	allowing others to help you	isolation
	EXERCISE:	helping others	selfish acts
	ELIMINATION:	forgiveness	temper tantrum

For an in depth study into "The Twelve Ingredients of Health" and the corresponding definition of Health I refer you to read the book titled Contract for a Healthy Life which is authored by my colleague and partner in crime, Cathy Hamill. In this book, she chronicles the genesis of these concepts, delves into their meaning and values. She also offers teaching materials and step by step guidelines for an incredible personal growth project. I highly recommend it!

How I connect our wellness terms to the habit *Sharpen the Saw* is first to address the fact that to perform at the most efficient and effective levels a person needs be mindful of all three areas of health. To become a successful and efficient person you need to maintain a state of wellness, but also to remain efficient and successful you must continually feed, rest, exercise and eliminate each area of health.

I explain that their own personal needs and goals may shift and require emphasis on one or more of the daily requirements more so than others from day to day, but balance is essential. I remind them that each area of health is interdependent and that includes both positive and negative aspects.

Keeping the body healthy, besides being worthwhile for its own sake, serves to maintain the energy levels required to achieve their project goal and other demands in their life. Undoubtedly, practicing the ability to reason and broaden understanding will lead to the most effective organization and planning of this project but also what is learned in the process of this project can be used for the success of future endeavors. The final part of the *Sharpen the Saw* habit concerns spiritual health. The relevancy of the emotional component is to take into account your feelings and personal purpose during this project and whether they support your life direction and relationships. In planning and reflection you need to ask yourself these questions; what did I learn from this project? what growth did I experience? and how did this project support social connections, my personal values and values of the greater good?

After making the connection to and reviewing the twelve ingredients of health, I ask them to think of someone they consider successful and ask them what they admire about that person. We talk some about what a successful life would look like. The typical things are said like; money, nice house, nice car, travel, etc. and then I ask them to ponder if that those are truly the measures of a successful life because it sounds kind of empty to me. I ask them to think about the successful person they had in mind and ask them how well this person fits into out model of wellness, are they a good example of how to balance all three areas of their health. Most times they admit the person that they had thought of was not a model example because often their lives would be out of balance by choosing work over family or physical wellness. I ask them if they feel Bill Gates would be considered successful. As the creator of Microsoft software and company he was a revolutionary and he could be said to have had an impact on each of us and the world. Yeah, we all agree that he is extremely successful! However, when he left his role as CEO of the company in 2008 it was to feed the parts of his life that he had neglected. His intellectual growth and development were constant and very productive. At the present time where he still has a role in the company but to a much lesser degree, Bill Gates works to balance his life better between work, his family and philanthropic projects. I would dare to say that he would say he is proud of the person he is today, and feels more successful than ever before.

Though I want my students to fully understand all the aspects of the habit *Sharpen the Saw*, my major emphasis with my middle school students regarding practicing of the habit *Sharpen the Saw* during this project is mostly about self-growth and reflection. I stress for them to choose a project that is something they have never done before or will push them out of their comfort zone in that by its design their experience will address this habit. I also alert them to the fact that at the end of their project they will need to complete a self-evaluation sheet. This forced reflective exercise asks that they assess their performances and feelings; as well as their physical, mental and spiritual growth.

To clarify this habit further, I go on to give examples from everyday life and ones that specifically relate to the project. One simply example I use is:

Jane felt very proud and appreciated after she served meals at the local Soup Kitchen. Going into this situation she never had been around homeless people before and had been somewhat nervous about it. She was not sure how they would treat her and how she should act around them. She had great pity for them but frankly was only doing this because she had to satisfy a community service requirement for school. While she served the people, many engaged her in conversations which helped her get over her initial shyness. They shared some very interesting stories about their life experiences and she ended up sharing a lot of laughs with them. Her allotted time flew by and was over before she knew it. In retrospect, Jane realized that these people were not scary at all. She found she enjoyed talking to them and would gladly come back to volunteer again.

We discuss as a class why it could be said that Jane demonstrates the habit, *Sharpen the Saw*. They initially come up with the fact that Jane celebrated her own accomplishments because she felt proud and appreciated. Where this is true she would have no doubt felt good and had pride about her selfless actions to better the day of less fortunate people. Yet it was her personal growth that really jumps out to me, the fact that she pushed herself beyond her "comfort zone" and gained new knowledge and insight as a result. Jane made real connections with people she would have never had otherwise. She changed previously formed opinions and attitudes to more open and considerate ones. I imagine that whether consciously or not that this is the major source of her pride.

Since this habit covers a lot of territory, I attempt to simplify how to begin practicing this habit by creating a list of personal qualities one could target to developing the habit. Some **keys to practicing this skill**, *Sharpen the Saw* are:

- ***To try new things***
- ***Explore and take healthy risks***
- ***Reflect upon new experiences and learning***
- ***Identify personal areas of growth***
- ***To be at peace and enjoy quiet moments***

My next step in class is to assess their understanding of the Habit: Sharpen the Saw. I do this by trying to have them make "real life" connections to our learning so far, I ask questions like:

What words might a person use to exhibit the habit Sharpen the Saw, can you give an example?
Can you think of a situation when you used this habit?
Can you think of person who often practices Sharpens the Saw, can you give examples of what they say or do?
Can you think of situation where someone used this habit or would have been better off if they had?
Can you think of a situation where you wish you had practiced Sharpening the Saw?

To further "hit home" the concept of *Sharpen the Saw* and how it can be practiced in this project I give a few examples of actual past student projects. I share stories about the students who did things that they never thought they could, and of learning and successes that were unexpected, and of students who were simply proud of accomplishing what they set out to do. Over time you will have examples of these stories to share with your students too. Here I will share one example taken directly from a student's poster. This young lady collected supplies and notes for US troops and donated them to the organization *Project from the Heart*. This organization sends the donations to US troops in Iraq and Afghanistan. She informed the school community via announcements and posters on the items she was collecting. She put a box in the cafeteria for one week and with permission from her homeroom teacher, her homeroom classmates were permitted to write letters to soldiers during the homeroom time slot. In all, she collected seventy-five letters and eight bags of supplies.

Habit 7: Sharpen the Saw

I didn't think about how much work people put into projects like this and how much they need and appreciate people helping them. Now I act more upon projects, for example when someone was collecting children's books, instead of ignoring it (like I used to), I wrote it down and brought in a bag full because now I know what it's like being the one collecting things. After doing this project, I am going to continue helping *Project from the Heart* outside of school. I plan to go to the IGA with my mom and set up a stand to collect money to help pay for sending the packages. We hope to be able to pay for one week of postage, which normally costs from $140-$185! I learned that you don't have to give a whole bunch to make a difference, and if everyone gave just a little, we would accomplish so much.

DESCRIBING THE PROJECT

The class after teaching the habits I review and probe for understanding of each habit. I use questions like the ones below to do this and to facilitate making a "real life" connection.

What words might a person use if they were using this habit, can you give an example?

Can you think of a situation where you did use this habit?

Can you think of person who often practices this habit, can you give examples of what they say or do?

Can you think of situation where someone used this habit or would have been better off if they had?

Can you think of a situation where you wish you had practiced that habit?

To expand upon their basic knowledge of the project parameters, I share some project themes and ideas of previous students and show them examples of exemplar student posters.

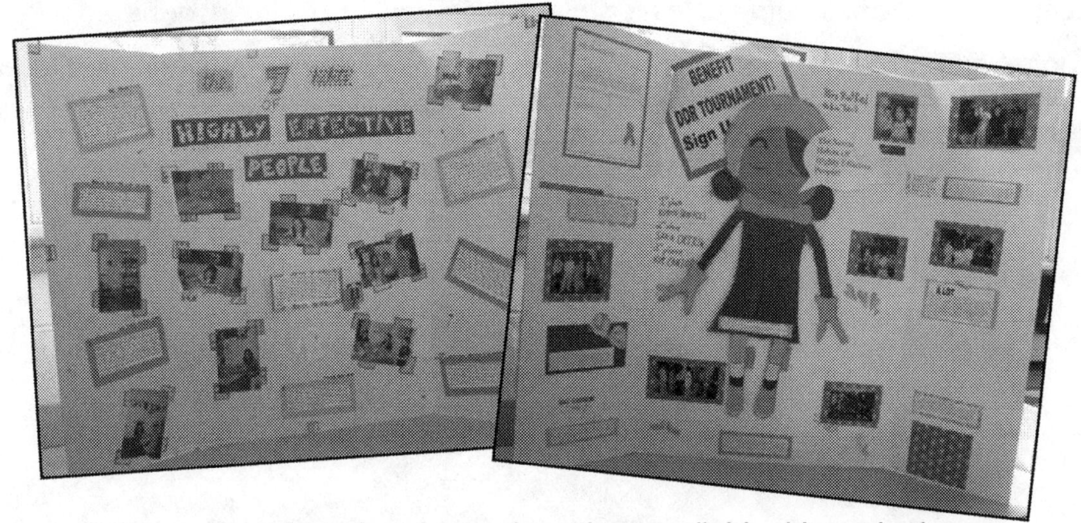

At times when there has been class time available, I have had my students complete an Inventory Packet to help them clarify a theme or idea for their own project. Sometimes due to time constraints I only distribute the Inventory Packet to be done by those who are struggling to come up with a project idea. I also have used the inventories as an aid for special education students to better understand the project and develop an idea. After having completed the inventories one of my students with Down Syndrome wasn't sure what to do for her project, I asked her about her Interest Inventory and she shared that she loves to draw fashion and hopes to be a fashion designer someday. Come to find out that she has pads full of drawings at home. As timing would have it, we were a few weeks from Mother's Day that year and she decided to compile her drawings along with a cover she made into a bound book for her mother. Her book along with a personal card turned out to be a cherished Mother's Day gift. The Inventory Packet and all the materials to which I will refer can be found in Chapter 6.

It is imperative for participants to come up with their own project idea. I made the mistake early on by suggesting an activity for a student and found his motivation, desire and drive was not that of the other students ... duh! They were following their personal drive toward a meaningful end and he was not. I learned my lesson! However, we sometimes guide our special education students to select project ideas that can be done in the school, during the school day so that their aide is able to offer guidance and/or assistance if needed. We try to limit adult involvement to scheduling time during the day and/or contacting the needed people if they have communication disabilities. Allowing them to be and feel in control and powerful is so important because often these of all students often are dependent upon adults and this often is the first activity independent of adult involvement (interference).

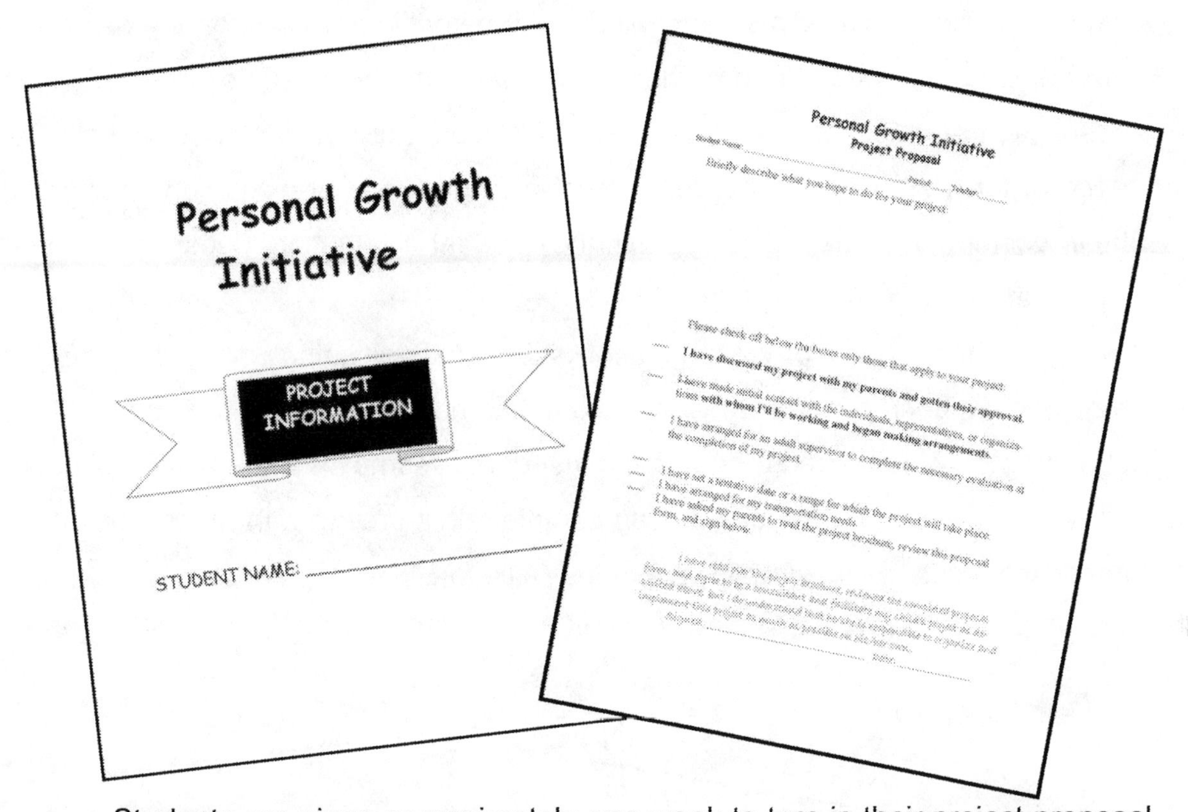

Students are given approximately one week to turn in their project proposal form. I suggest reviewing the proposals and returning them to students quickly so they can get to work, or have time to change in the event of something falling through. Where I have never had to "reject" a project proposal, I may ask the student to reevaluate the feasibility of what is being proposed I either do this face to face or by writing questions on the proposal to help them better define their thinking, such as; do you know how many times will you be doing this?, where?, when?, how long will you do it? Where I prefer students to do an individual project, there have been occasions were students devise a way to work together that will still afford each participant to practice all the habits. For example they both wish to go to a convalescent home at the same time but one partner will be playing a concert for the patients and the other has baked and organized refreshments for them to enjoy after the concert. Their approach requires both parties to have made the necessary contacts, planned and organized resources as if having done an individual project.

I give them approximately six weeks to complete their task and create a visual presentation. In addition to a poster, the other written assignments include a student evaluation and an adult evaluation sheet which are due on the same day as the poster. I require that the poster have a title, visuals, and a project description. It must also name and give an account of how well he/she practiced each of the seven habits. Students must also give oral presentations describing their posters and their answers on the student evaluation questions to their classmates.

Full size copies of the evaluation sheets, poster guidelines and the project rubrics have been provided in Chapter 6. I also have included modified evaluation sheets and poster rubrics that I have used with some of my special education students, however most students can complete this project with few modifications because by nature it easily allows for differentiation.

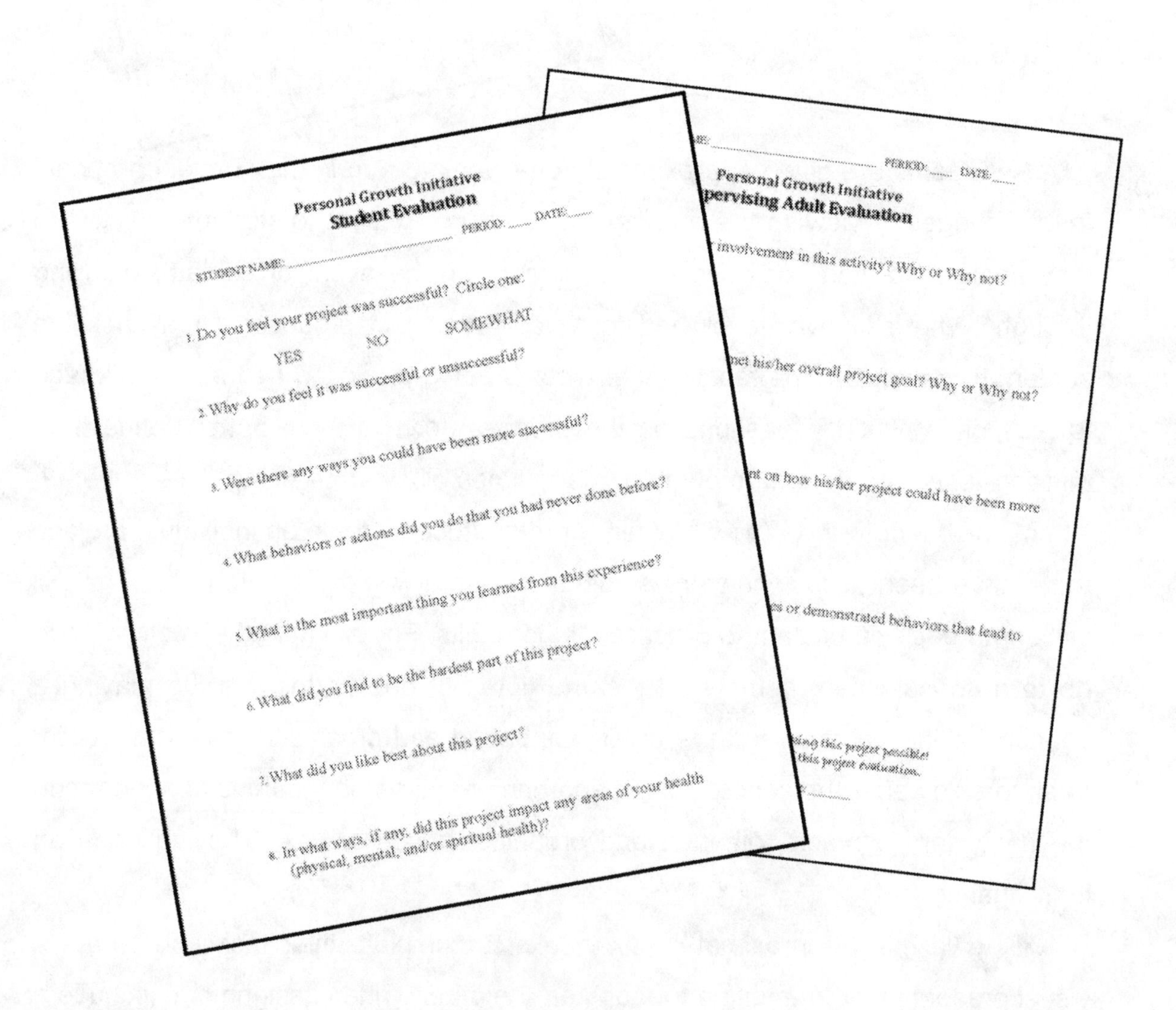

Personal Growth Initiative
Student Evaluation

STUDENT NAME: ____________ PERIOD: ___ DATE: ___

1. Do you feel your project was successful? Circle one:

YES NO SOMEWHAT

2. Why do you feel it was successful or unsuccessful?

3. Were there any ways you could have been more successful?

4. What behaviors or actions did you do that you had never done before?

5. What is the most important thing you learned from this experience?

6. What did you find to be the hardest part of this project?

7. What did you like best about this project?

8. In what ways, if any, did this project impact any areas of your health (physical, mental, and/or spiritual health)?

Personal Growth Initiative
pervising Adult Evaluation

involvement in this activity? Why or Why not?

met his/her overall project goal? Why or Why not?

nt on how his/her project could have been more

s or demonstrated behaviors that lead to

Chapter 5: REPRODUCIBLE MATERIALS

Project Brochure

Inventory Packet:

Interests Inventory, Character Traits Inventory, Personality Inventory, Wrap-up

Project Packet #1:

Project Synopsis
Overview of the 7 Habits
Project Proposal
Planning Sheet

Classroom and Home Activities:

Activity Directions
Identifying the 7 Habits Worksheet
Identifying the 7 Habits Answer Sheet

Project Packet #2:

Review of the 7 Habits
Project Rubric
Reflection Questions
Sample Poster Caption Write-up
Student Evaluation
Adult Evaluation

Printout PowerPoint Slide Show:

Introduction to the Project and 7 Habits

Modified Packet

Grade 7

Personal Growth Innitiative

7 Habits of Highly Effective People Project

Due: ______

REQUIRED WRITTEN ASSIGNMENTS

~ Project Proposal

~ Student Evaluation Form

~ Supervising Adult Evaluation Form

FINAL PRESENTATION

POSTER &

VERBAL

PRESENTATION

PROJECT DESCRIPTION

The student will put Stephen Covey's Habits of Highly Effective People into practice in an individualized project.

The student will choose an activity or a series of activities that you must initiate, organize and implement.

Stephen Covey's Seven Habits of Highly Effective People

Habit 1: BE PROACTIVE
"You= The Programmer"

Habit 2: BEGIN WITH THE END IN MIND
"The Program"

Habit 3: PUT FIRST THINGS FIRST
"Personal Management"

Habit 4: THINK WIN-WIN
"Mutual Benefit"

Habit 5: SEEK FIRST TO UNDERSTAND, THEN TO BE UNDERSTOOD
"True Communication"

Habit 6: SYERGIZE
"Creative Cooperation"

Habit 7: SHARPEN THE SAW
"Personal Growth"

YOUR PERSONAL GROWTH INITIATIVE

Inventory Packet

The following inventories are designed to get you thinking about who you are and what types of activities would be best suited to your interests, values and personality.

You are more likely to be satisfied and successful if your choice of activity is something that you have never tried before, will excite you and be fun!

Here you go...

Interests Inventory

Read through each selection put a check in front of the areas you would say are high interests of yours. That is that you enjoy doing, want to learn more about and/or may want to do when you grow up.

☐ MUSIC

☐ ART

☐ WRITING (journalism, poetry or short stories)

☐ ENTERTAINMENT (drama, comedy, magic, dance)

☐ COMPUTERS

☐ MEDIA GAMES (computer, TV)

☐ PHOTOGRAPHY (photos, video, film)

☐ ANIMALS (domestic, wild)

☐ PUBLIC SERVICE (politics, medicine, social work)

☐ TEACHING (academic, sports)

☐ CHILD CARE

☐ ENVIRONMENT (ecology, recycling, resource protection)

☐ TECHNOLOGY (mechanical, electrical, engineering)

☐ COOKING

☐ SPORTS/FITNESS

☐ LAW ENFORCEMENT/ MILITARY (want to protect and defend)

☐ BUSINESS/INDUSTRY (yard work, babysitting, car washing, dog walking)

List below what you would consider your top 3 areas of interest either currently or you might want to part of your adult life.

1.______________________________

2.______________________________

3.______________________________

Character Traits Inventory

Read through each selection put a check in front of the areas you would say you currently exemplify or would most like to exemplify. You can choose a trait you might not feel you demonstrate yet, but wish to work on developing it.

- ☐ ADVOCACY (teach others about causes or beliefs)
- ☐ CARING (kindness, generosity)
- ☐ CITIZENSHIP (patriotism, community service)
- ☐ COMMUNICATION (effective speaking and listening)
- ☐ CONSERVATION (ecology, preservation)
- ☐ EMPATHY (compassion, concern for others)
- ☐ HEALTH (being physically, mentally, and emotionally happy)
- ☐ IMAGINATION (creative, inventive)
- ☐ LEADERSHIP (setting a good example, taking charge)
- ☐ RELATIONSHIPS (positive interactions with family, friends and others)
- ☐ RESPONSIBILITY (dependability, reliability)
- ☐ RESPECT (polite, considerate, reverent)
- ☐ SAFETY (aware of danger, prevent harm)
- ☐ WISDOM (knowledge, common sense)
- ☐ PEACEFULNESS (cooperative, good conflict resolution skills)
- ☐ PURPOSE (focused, driven by goals)

List below what you would consider to be the top 3 traits that you would like to exemplify in your daily life, now or in the future.

1.______________________________
2.______________________________
3.______________________________

Personality Inventory

Read through each selection put a check in front the personality traits that are most like you. The statements you are most likely to feel or most like they way you would behave.

OPINIONS

_____ I am usually comfortable sharing my view points and opinions at home.
_____I am usually comfortable sharing my viewpoints and opinions at school.
_____I am rarely comfortable sharing my viewpoints and opinions.

ROLE MODELS

_____ I have older people I look to for advice and guidance.
_____Younger people look to me sometimes for advice and help.
_____ I don't really have any role models in my life.

CONFIDENCE

_____ When faced with something new, I think I can do it if I try my best.
_____I panic when faced with something new and initially I think I can't do it.

LEARNING STYLES

_____ I come up with good ideas. I am very creative and like to problem solve.
_____I like to work hard with a set routine and schedule. I like knowing what to expect when I'm done.

GOALS

_____I tend to procrastinate… I put things off until it's nearly or is too late.
_____I tend to make a plan for myself and follow it step by step until I'm done.
_____If someone sets up a schedule for me, I'll stick to it and get things done.

RESPONSIBILITY

_____ I can take charge and organize other people and things to meet assigned deadlines.
_____I am forgetful and may be late in getting to places or finishing tasks.
_____I do not see the importance of sticking to deadlines, if I get it done that is what is important.

FAMILY

_____ I enjoy and spend a good amount of time with my parents and family.
_____I wish I could spend more time with my parents and family.
_____My parents want me to spend more time with the family, but I'd rather not.

RISK TAKING

_____ I usually will try new things, even if I'm not sure I'll succeed.
_____I'll try something new if I'm pretty sure I'm going to be good at it.
_____I have some great ideas but could never get myself to try them.

Personal Growth Initiative Inventory Wrap-up: Pg.1

"Putting it all together"

The Why and How... (GOALS)

Read through each selection. Put a check at the selections that could be a goal that could excite and motivate you.

_____ I want to make a difference to another person (face to face)

_____ I want to make a difference to a group or community

_____ I want to create something

_____ I want to improve something

_____ I want to make a change or improve myself

The Who and What... (ACTIVITIES &TOPICS)

ACTIVITIES: Read through each selection. Put a check at the selections that could be an activity that could excite and motivate you.

_____ I want to find a way to utilize a skill or talent of mine

_____ I want to teach a skill

_____ I want to plan an event... party, dinner, a family or friend gathering or outing

_____ I want to collect money, clothes, books, food, etc and donate to a cause or charity

_____ I want to educate others: provide needed information or publicize a cause or need

_____ I want to make a change or improve my current behaviors

_____ I want to learn a skill

Personal Growth Initiative Inventory Wrap-up: Pg. 2

TOPICS: Read through each selection. Put a check at topics you feel are most important to you. I f you have marked off more than five, go back and circle the top 5.

_____ animal care and welfare

_____ environmental issues

_____ fitness/sports

_____ fight against hunger

_____ promote literacy

_____ politics (local, state, national)

_____ humor/fun

_____ help the homeless

_____ help the elderly

_____ help the sick and injured

_____ work with children

_____ your family

_____ prevent abuse and violence

_____ school (staff, students, building, clubs, activities)

_____ help the underprivileged (those who have less than you)

_____ tolerance & equality (fairness to all races and genders)

_____ help the disabled (physically, mentally)

_____ wellness (promote healthy living, disease prevention and charities)

_____ religion/culture (practice your faith, share and teach your beliefs and customs)

_____ personal improvement (your fitness, diet, study habits, stress/anger management, relationshi

While completing these inventories did you get a brilliant idea?

If yes, check with the necessary people for approval and to work out details and then fill out your project proposal form and get started.

If no, review the inventories for themes and ways to put some your interests and skills to use. You can also share your inventories with a close friend, parent or teacher to see if anyone has an idea that you ultimately believe you would find fun and meaningful. Then check with the necessary people for approval and to work out details and then fill out your project proposal form and get started.

NOW, GO DO GREAT THINGS AND ENJOY!

Personal Growth Initiative

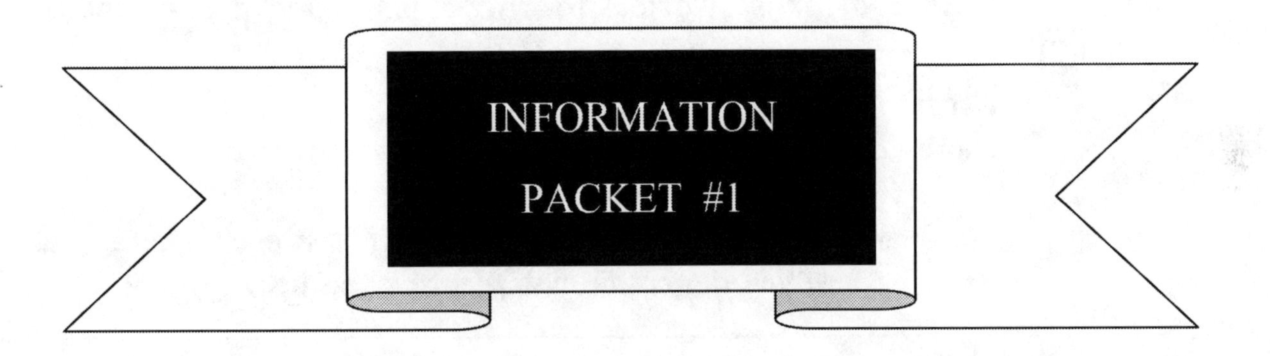

STUDENT NAME: ______________________________

Personal Growth Initiative
Project Requirements

Action: Plan and complete an activity that will allow you to practice the 7 Habits of Highly Effective People.

Required Written Assignments:

- ✓ Project Proposal
- ✓ Supervising Adult Evaluation
- ✓ Student Evaluation Form

Project Poster and Oral Presentation:

You will create a poster that teaches about your project and shows your understanding of Steven Covey's 7 Habits of Highly Effective People. Finally, you will explain your project and poster in an oral presentation to the class. Your poster must include:

- **A title**
- **Photos and/or visuals that teach about your project**
- **A brief description of your project**
- **The names of all 7 Habits and a caption for each where you describe how you did or did not practice the habit.**

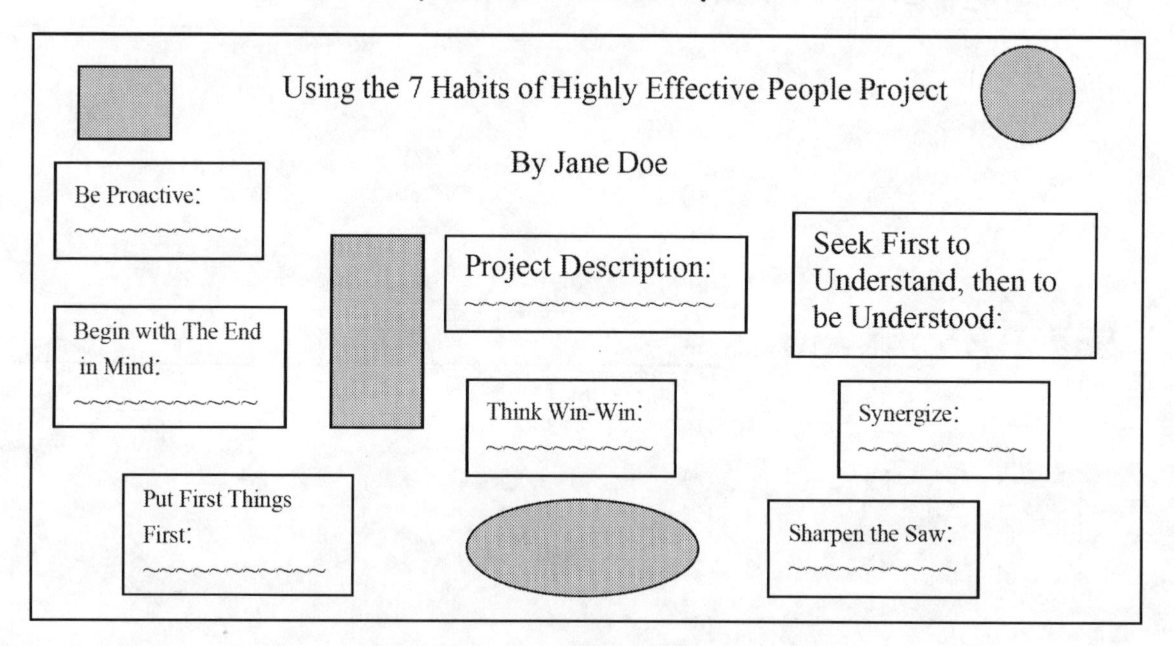

The Seven Habits of Highly Effective People Overview

Habit 1 Be Proactive

« Take responsibility for your actions »

Habit Defined: Proactive means taking initiative, not waiting for others to act first, and being responsible for what you do. The opposite of proactive is reactive. Reactive people act in response to what goes on around them (couch potatoes) and act without conviction or purpose. The actions of proactive people are deliberate and purposely based upon their principles and values.

Keys to practicing the skills:

⇒ Know yourself and what you feel is worthy of your energy and time

⇒ The ability to make and keep commitments and promises is at the heart of this habit

⇒ Understand possible consequences and mistakes

Synonyms:

Innovative

Responsible

Purposeful

Visionary

Example: Since Joe's mother has gone back to working at nights he finds that she is often tired, stressed and cranky in the mornings. He tells her that from now on he'll make breakfast each morning for him and his sister so she can sleep late.

Habit 2 Begin With The End in Mind

« Determine your goal before you »

Habit Defined: Begin With The End in Mind means to begin with the image of what you want to happen so you can use it as a frame of reference to measure your progress. This is the mental preparation that needs to occur before any physical action takes place.

Keys to practicing the skills:

⇒ Think first, before you act

⇒ Visualize what you want the outcome to be or the way you want something to turn out

Synonyms:

Vision

Mission

Design

Mental Creation

Mental Preparation

Example: Liz wants to have a Halloween party for her friends. She wants everyone to come to her house in costume so they can trick or treat in her neighborhood. When it starts to get late they can go back to her house to watch a scary movie and sort their candy.

Habit 3 Put First Things First

<< Prioritize, and do the first things first> >

Habit Defined: To Put First Things First means to create a plan of action to achieve your personal mission and not compromise the other areas in your life. Strive to preserve a proper balance in your life by prioritizing and doing the most important things first.

Keys to practicing the skills:

⇒ List the "to dos" by priority
⇒ Create a checklist of what needs to be done
⇒ Use a calendar or long term planner to track progress

Synonyms:

Discipline
Planning
Organization
Personal Management

Example: Kelsey first called the animal shelter to see what kind of donations they would want or need. After asking her parents when they could drive her to the shelter she checked her personal calendar then she set a collection date and put all the details on flyers that she put in her neighbors' mailboxes.

Habit 4 Think Win-Win

<< Think of mutually benefit >>

Habit Defined: To Think Win/Win means to seek those situations, solutions, projects, and relationships that are mutually satisfying. When you come upon a problem, you are optimistic when trying to solve it and know when you walk away from it that you still learned something from it.

Keys to practicing the skills:

⇒ Think "we", not "I"
⇒ When you can't achieve a "win/win" deal, accept that agreeing to disagree may be the best you can do
⇒ Compromise if necessary for both involved to get something they wanted progress
⇒ Be positive when faced with a problem and try to make any change for the better

Synonyms:

Respectful
Positive
Cooperative
Considerate
Flexible

Example: Tom's mother asks him to clean out his closet and get rid of all his clothes that he has outgrown. He suggests that he should bag all the clothes and donate them to a clothing drive at school for the local homeless shelter. His mother agrees about the donating the clothes and after she sees how empty his closet is and suggests that she take him shopping soon for new clothes.

Habit 5 Seek First to Understand, Then to Be Understood

« Ask questions to fully understand and listen sincerely to people »

Habit Defined: Seek First to Understand, Then to Be Understood means to listen with genuine interest to fully understand both the feeling and meaning of the other person's words. Effective communication is taking into account the perspective of that person in creating your response and then clearly sharing your thoughts and/or expectations.

Keys to practicing the skills:

⇒ Ask questions to clarify that you understand correctly

⇒ Probe for further meaning, tone, body language, etc.

⇒ Present your ideas and needs clearly, and specifically as they relate to the listener

Synonyms:

Perceptive
Empathetic
Articulate
Good Communicator

Example: Before choosing a book and activity to do on her visit to a 2nd grade class, Susie contacted the teacher and asked if there was a topic her students were especially interested in, or a topic the teacher would like her to teach.

Habit 6 Synergize:

«Work with others. Cooperate »

Habit Defined: Synergize means to work with others, cooperate, and be open to new ideas or ways. Through mutual trust and understanding problems can be solved and ideas created that are obtained through a joining of individual ideas and strengths.

Keys to practicing the skills:

⇒ Ask for input or new insights from others

⇒ Seek new alternatives, brainstorm with others for different solutions

Synonyms:

Open Minded
Cooperative
Collaborative
Alternative Seeking

Example: Brian has collected a lot of books to donate to an elementary school that does not have many classroom libraries. The elementary school principal suggests that when he drops off the books to the school that he should stay and read one of his favorite books to one of the classes. After reading his story to the class, he got to see the joy the children were experiencing while exploring their new books.

Habit 7 Sharpen the Saw

« Reflect and rejuvenate »

Habit Defined: Sharpen the Saw means to take time to reflect and rejuvenate. This sharpening allows for personal growth and change. Giving yourself credit for what you did well, and forgiving yourself for any mistakes. This habit promotes continuous balancing of one's mental, physical and spiritual health.

Keys to practicing the skills:

⇒ Try something new
⇒ Explore and take healthy risks
⇒ Reflect on new experiences and learning
⇒ Identify personal area of growth

Synonyms:

Self Renewal
Replenish
Recharge
Personal Growth

Example: Jay felt very proud and appreciated after he served meals at Operation Hope. He never had been around homeless people and was somewhat frightened, yet after getting over his initial shyness he found he really enjoyed talking to them, they were not scary, and they shared a lot of laughs.

Personal Growth Initiative

Project Proposal

Student Name: ______________________________ Period: ____ Teacher:_______

1. Briefly describe what you hope to do for your project:

2. What aspect of this activity will you be doing for the first time?

3. Please **check off** below **only those boxes that apply to you and your project**:

☐ I have discussed my project with my parents and gotten their approval.

☐ I have made initial contact with the individuals, representatives, or organizations with whom I'll be working and began making arrangements.

☐ I have set a tentative date or a range for which the project will take place.

☐ I have begun arranging for any resources or transportation needs.

☐ I have arranged for an adult supervisor to complete the necessary evaluation at the completion of my project.

☐ I have asked my parents to read the project brochure, review this proposal form, and will sign below.

I have read over the project brochure, reviewed the completed proposal form, and agree to be a consultant and facilitate my child's project as described above, but I do understand that he/she is responsible to organize and implement this project as much as possible on his/her own.

Signed: ______________________________ Date: ______________

Personal Growth Initiative
Planning Sheet

Student Name: ______________________________

Directions:

1. List in the first column all the tasks you believe you need to accomplish to make your project a success; steps to take, resources needed, contacts needed, etc. You can add to this list if new ideas come to you after you begin.
2. In the second column break this list by priority; urgent or necessary.

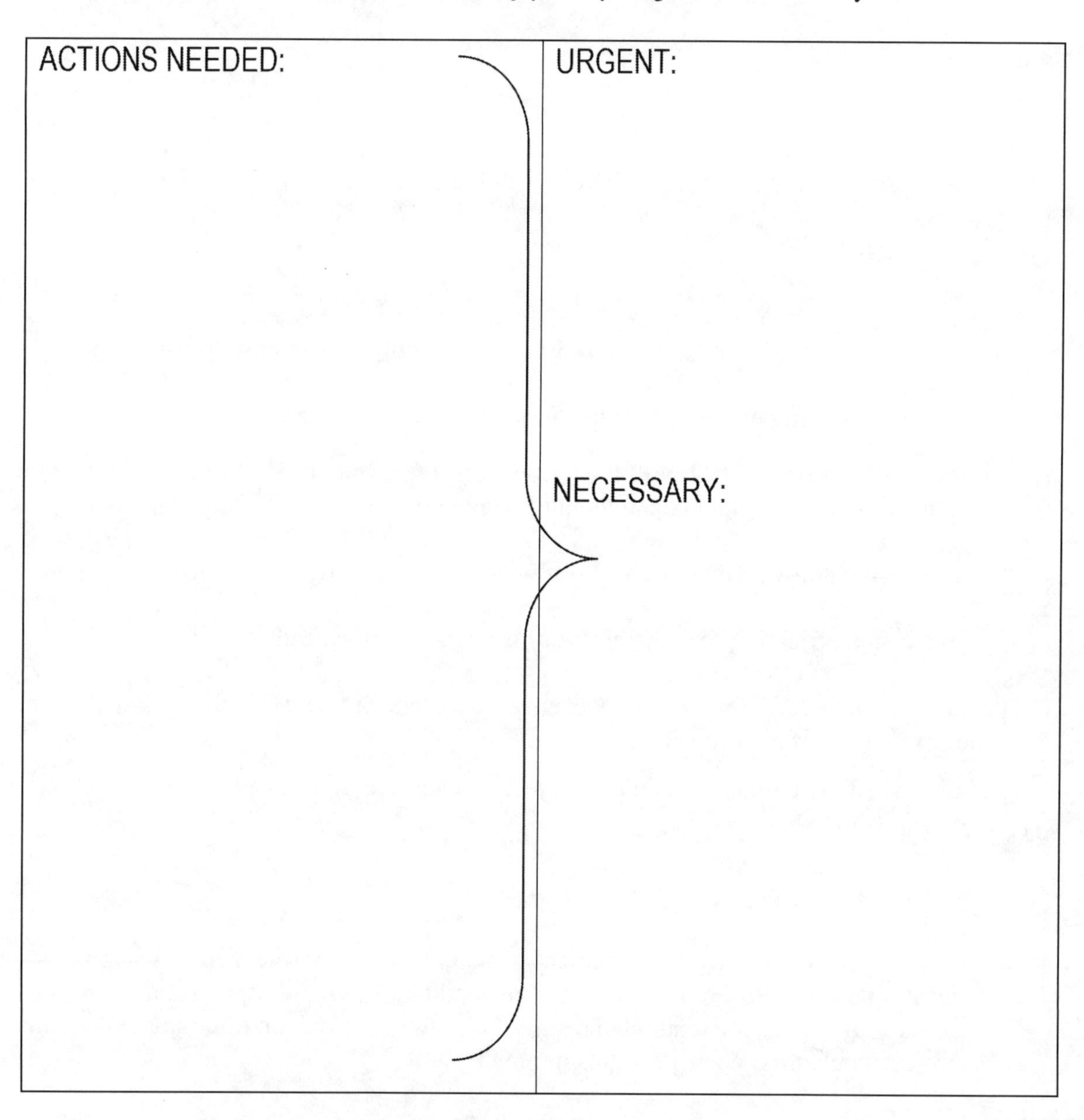

Can you identify the 7 Habits of Highly Effective People?

WORKSHEET DIRECTIONS

This assignment can be used in class or as a homework assignment.

- Distribute the worksheets to individuals or pairs of students to assess their understanding of the 7 Habits of Highly Effective People.
- Answer Sheet offers the answers and bolded key phrases to differentiate why the habit was selected.

Worksheet Directions: **Identify which of the 7 Habits is most demonstrated in each scenario. Write the name of the habit in the blank after each scenario. Each habit will have only one match.**

ALTERNATIVE ACTIVITY & DIRECTIONS

These days, more often than using the worksheet I cut the scenarios up separately and put the & habits on small separate pieces of paper and have the students do a matching card game.

- Distribute 7 scenarios cards and 7 cards each with one name of a Habit.
- Individually or in pairs the students match a scenario with the name of the Habit that is most demonstrated in that scenario.
- Answer Sheet offers the answers and highlights the key phrases to differentiate why the habit was selected.

Can you identify the 7 Habits of Highly Effective People?

STUDENT NAME: ______________________________ PERIOD: ___

Directions: Identify which of the 7 Habits is most demonstrated in each scenario. Write the name of the habit in the blank after each scenario. Each habit will have only one match.

Jay felt very proud and appreciated after he served meals at Operation Hope. He never had been around homeless people and was somewhat frightened, yet after getting over his initial shyness he found he really enjoyed talking to them, they were not scary, and they shared a lot of laughs.	________
Before choosing a book and activity to do on her visit to a 2nd grade class, Susie contacted the teacher and asked if there was a topic her students were especially interested in, or a topic the teacher would like her to teach. Then she chose a book to read to the class.	________
Since Joe's mother has gone back to working at nights he finds that she is often tired, stressed and cranky in the mornings. He tells her that from now on he'll make breakfast each morning for him and his sister so she can sleep late.	________
Kelsey first called the animal shelter to see what kind of donations they would want or need. After asking her parents when they could drive her to the shelter, she set a collection date and put all the details on flyers that she put in her neighbor's mailboxes.	________
Tom's mother asks him to clean out his closet and get rid of all his clothes that he has outgrown so he can fit new ones. He suggests that he should bag all the clothes and donate them to the needy.	________
Liz wants to have a Halloween party for her friends. She wants everyone to come to her house in costume so they can trick or treat in her neighborhood. When it starts to get late they can all go back to her house to watch a scary movie and sort their candy.	________
Brian has collected a lot of books to donate to an elementary school that does not have many classroom libraries and calls to schedule a time to drop them off. The principal suggests that when he drops off the books to the school that he should stay and read one of his favorite books to one of the classes. After reading his story to the class, he got to see the joy the children had exploring their new books.	________

Can you identify the 7 Habits of Highly Effective People?

ANSWER SHEET

Jay **felt very proud and appreciated** after he served meals at Operation Hope. He never had been around homeless people and was somewhat frightened, **yet after getting over his initial shyness he found he really enjoyed talking to them, they were not scary**, and they shared a lot of laughs.	**SHARPEN THE SAW**
Before choosing a book and activity to do on her visit to a 2nd grade class, **Susie contacted the teacher and asked** if there was a topic her students were especially interested in, or a topic the teacher would like her to teach. Then she chose a book to read to the class.	**SEEK FIRST TO UNDERSTAND, THEN TO BE UNDERSTOOD**
Since Joe's mother has gone back to working at nights he finds that she is often tired, stressed and cranky in the mornings. **He tells her** that from now on he'll make breakfast each morning for him and his sister so she can sleep late.	**BE PROACTIVE**
Kelsey **first called the animal shelter** to see what kind of donations they would want or need. **After asking her parents** when they could drive her to the shelter, she **set a collection date** and **put all the details on flyers** that she **put in her neighbor's mailboxes.**	**PUT FIRST THINGS FIRST**
Tom's mother asks him to clean out his closet and get rid of all his clothes that he has outgrown so he can fit new ones. **He suggests that he should bag all the clothes and donate them to the needy.**	**THINK WIN-WIN**
Liz wants to have a Halloween party for her friends. She wants everyone to **come to her house in costume** so they can **trick or treat in her neighborhood**. When it starts to get late they can all **go back to her house to watch a scary movie** and **sort their candy.**	**BEGIN WITH THE END IN MIND**
Brian has collected a lot of books to donate to an elementary school that does not have many classroom libraries. **The principal suggests** that when he drops off the books to the school that **he should stay and read** one of his favorite books to one of the classes. **After reading his story to the class**, he got to see the joy the children had exploring their new books.	**SYNERGIZE**

Personal Growth Initiative

PROJECT
INFORMATION
PACKET #2

STUDENT NAME: ______________________________

PROJECT DUE: __________

Personal Growth Initiative

Project Requirements

Action: Plan and complete an activity that will allow you to practice the 7 Habits of Highly Effective People.

Required Written Assignments:

- ✓ Project Proposal
- ✓ Supervising Adult Evaluation
- ✓ Student Evaluation Form

Project Poster and Oral Presentation:

You will create a poster that teaches about your project and shows your understanding of Steven Covey's 7 Habits of Highly Effective People. Finally, you will explain your project and poster in an oral presentation to the class. Your poster must include:

- **A title**
- **Photos and/or visuals that teach about your project**
- **A brief description of your project**
- **The names of all 7 Habits and a caption for each where you describe how you did or did not practice the habit.**

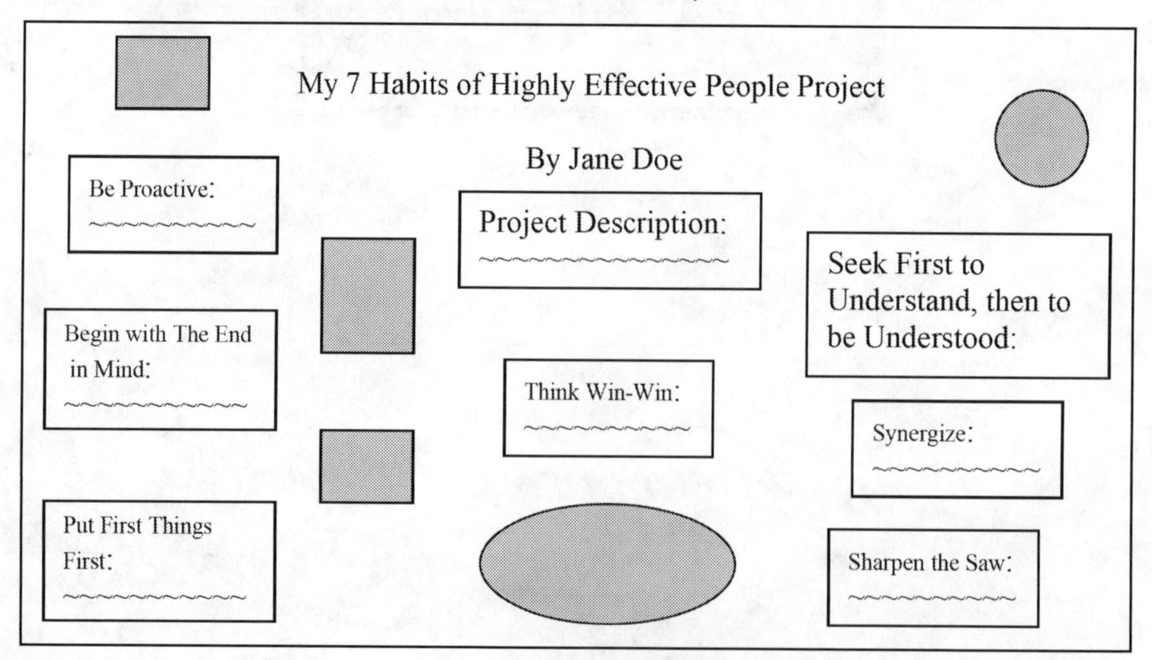

Personal Growth Initiative Grading Sheet

STUDENT NAME:________________________ PERIOD:____ DATE:____

ORAL PRESENTATION

RUBRIC AND POINT EARNINGS

AREA	AWESOME	ACCEPTABLE	MINIMAL	UNACCEPTABLE
Content	Clearly overviewed project, reason for choosing it, and project's goal	Described project and goal	Some explanation of project	Little to no project description
Delivery	Clear voice, loud, and pleasant Showed confidence, comfort and high degree of understanding. and preparation	Adequate voice tone and volume Appeared confident and prepared.	Low voice quality and showed little confidence and effort.	Voice tone or volume took away from delivery. Showed little to no evidence of preparation
	(15-20 points)	(10-15 points)	(5-10 points)	(0-5 points)

ORAL PRESENTATION = _____ POINTS

VISUAL PRESENTATION= _____ POINTS

TOTAL POINTS= _____

FINAL GRADE=

Personal Growth Initiative Grading Sheet Pg.2

VISUAL PRESENTATION

POSTER RUBRIC AND POINT EARNINGS

AREA	AWESOME	ACCEPTABLE	MINIMAL	UNACCEPTABLE
Content	Well-written labels captions that illustrate and inform about the meaningful project, application of the 7 Habits and impact on personal wellness. (50-60 points)	Captions that inform viewer about the project, the 7 Habits and impact on wellness. (40-50 points)	Captions inform minimally or are incomplete about the required topics. (30-40 points)	Text is non-existent, incomplete, inaccurate, or fail to inform (0-30 points)
Design	Layout contains appropriate photos or visuals that are easily read, logical and neat. (8-10 points)	Layout contains photos, is mostly neat, fairly logical and easy to understand . (6-8 points)	Somewhat disorganized; and hard to understand. (4-6 points)	Disorganized; appears unplanned and done hastily. (1-3 points)
Visual	Visuals capture viewer's attention and interest and are effective. (4-5 points)	Good use of color and eye-catching elements (3-4 points)	Some good ideas but something detracts from the message. (2-3 points)	Color, photos or graphic details minimal or poorly done. (1-2 points)
Creativity	Unique ideas, and/or design making the poster stand-out. (4-5 points)	Contains some unique, original, or imaginative ideas. (3-4 points)	Some good creativity. (2-3 points)	Little or no evidence of creativity. (1-2 points)

Personal Growth Initiative

REFLECTION QUESTIONS:

Use these questions to help you write your explanation about how you practiced each of the 7 habits of Highly Effective people.

Habit 1 Be Proactive < Take responsibility for your actions ...

- WHY DID I FEEL MY ACTIVITY OR GOAL WAS IMPORTANT FOR ME TO DO? WHY WAS IT VALUABLE?
- BEFORE I STARTED, WHICH ACTIONS AND THOUGHTS MADE ME THINK I WAS GOING TO BE SUCCESSFUL?
- WAS I RESPONSIBLE? DID I KEEP MY COMMITMENTS?

Habit 2 Begin With The End in Mind: < your project goal ...

- DID I HAVE A CLEAR PICTURE OF WHAT I WANTED TO HAPPEN BEFORE I STARTED?
- DID IT TURN OUT THE WAY I HAD PLANNED?
- DID I ACCOMPLISH MY GOAL?

Habit 3 Put First Things First: < Prioritize, and organize steps to take...

- WHAT ORGANIZATIONAL STEPS DID I TAKE?
- DID I CHANGE MY SCHEDULE OR PUT OFF OTHER THINGS TO MAKE IT HAPPEN?

Habit 4 **Think Win-Win:** ‹ Be optimistic... don't get down by problems...

- DID I HAVE A POSITIVE ATTITUDE?
- DID THIS ACTIVITY BENEFIT OTHERS AS WELL AS ME?
- DID A PROBLEM COME UP THAT I WORKED OUT CALMLY WITH A POSITIVE RESULT?

Habit 5 **Seek First to Understand, Then to Be Understood**

‹ Ask questions to fully understand and listen sincerely to people...

- DID I LISTEN TO FIND OUT WHAT OTHER'S FELT AND NEEDED?
- DID I MAKE IT CLEAR TO THE OTHER PEOPLE WHAT I PLANNED TO DO?

Habit 6 **Synergize:** ‹ Collaboration - Working with others. ...

- HOW DID I WORK WITH OTHERS?
- DID I LISTEN TO OTHER PEOPLE'S SUGGESTIONS?
- DID I USE ANY IDEAS FROM OTHER PEOPLE?

Habit 7 **Sharpen the Saw:** ‹ Reflection- Growth...

- WHAT DID I TRY THAT I NEVER HAD DONE BEFORE?
- HOW WELL DID I DO?
- WHAT CAN I LEARN FROM THIS?

A Written Sample of A Student Linking His Project To The "7 Habits"

Project Description:

I taught a 7 year old neighbor some skateboarding tricks. We had four hour long practices and I taught him the following skateboarding tricks; ride on the ground, go down a flat ramp, go up and down a sloped ramp, drop in on a flat ramp, turn around on a flat ramp and in a halfpipe.

Habit One: Be Proactive

I chose a project that was fun and enjoyable, but also was something I could stick with to the end. I like skateboarding and knew I could keep the commitment required to teach someone else.

Habit Two: Begin with the End in Mind

I wanted to be able to teach a younger kid some basic skateboarding skills at the skate park. I wanted my student to be old enough to concentrate and be motivated to work hard for about an hour. I hoped with four practice sessions he could learn three or four tricks.

Habit Three: Put First Things First

First I had to find out that it was O.K. with my parents. Then I had to find someone to teach. I called the mother of a neighbor that I knew wanted to learn to skateboard and asked if it would be O.K. We figured out and made plans for the days that would work out for both of us. Lastly, I had to think of how and what I would be teaching him. Once I had all the dates and was sure to have a ride to the skating park, I still had to make a list of what I was going to teach and how. I made a list of tricks I thought a 7 year old could master and brought it with me each time.

Habit Four: Think Win-Win

When my student fell, got stuck or couldn't do a trick I tried to encourage him. I gave him more tips and tried harder to help him learn it. I tried to discourage his competitive attitude. I explained as long as he tried his best, and didn't get discouraged he would pick up more and get it sooner.

Habit Five: Seek first to Understand, Then to be Understood

When starting this project I had to be sure that this would be something the child would enjoy and really want to do. I had to listen to not only to what he had to say, but also his mother's opinions. I had to make it clear to him that it might be hard and frustrating, but he had to be willing to commit to a certain number of hours for us to have success and me to complete my project. If I had not he and his mother may have had been expecting something to happen that didn't, or not expected something that I had wanted to do.

Habit Six: Synergize

There were times when he saw a trick being done by another skateboarder and asked if he could learn it, so a few times we added those tricks to the list of skills. Other times I had to explain that he needed to learn other tricks first, and that the trick would be too dangerous for him to try. So, I feel it was good for me not to have stick to my original list of tricks and to have added his choices too, because he learned tricks that I hadn't thought of and ones he really wanted to learn.

Habit Seven: Sharpen the Saw

When I chose this project, I wanted it to develop my skateboarding skills and it did, but I think it helped in other ways as well. It helped me in "working with others'. It helped me with "communication skills": listening and explaining things.

Personal Growth Initiative

Student Evaluation

STUDENT NAME: ______________________________ PERIOD: ___ DATE:___

1. Do you feel your project was successful? Circle one:

   YES NO SOMEWHAT

2. Why do you feel it was successful or unsuccessful?

3. Were there any ways you could have been more successful?

4. What behaviors or actions did you do that you had never done before?

5. What is the most important thing you learned from this experience?

6. What did you find to be the hardest part of this project?

7. What did you like best about this project?

8. In what ways, if any, did this project impact any areas of your health (physical, mental, and/or spiritual health)?

STUDENT NAME: ______________________________ PERIOD: ___ DATE: ____

Personal Growth Initiative

Supervising Adult Evaluation

1. Did you enjoy your involvement in this activity? Why or Why not?

2. Do you feel the student met his/her overall project goal? Why or Why not?

3. Any suggestions for the student on how his/her project could have been more successful?

4. Can you name any personal attributes or demonstrated behaviors that lead to his/her success?

Thank you for your time and effort in making this project possible! Please sign below to verify the completion of this project evaluation.

Signature: _____________________________ ***Print Name:*** ________________

Personal Growth Initiative

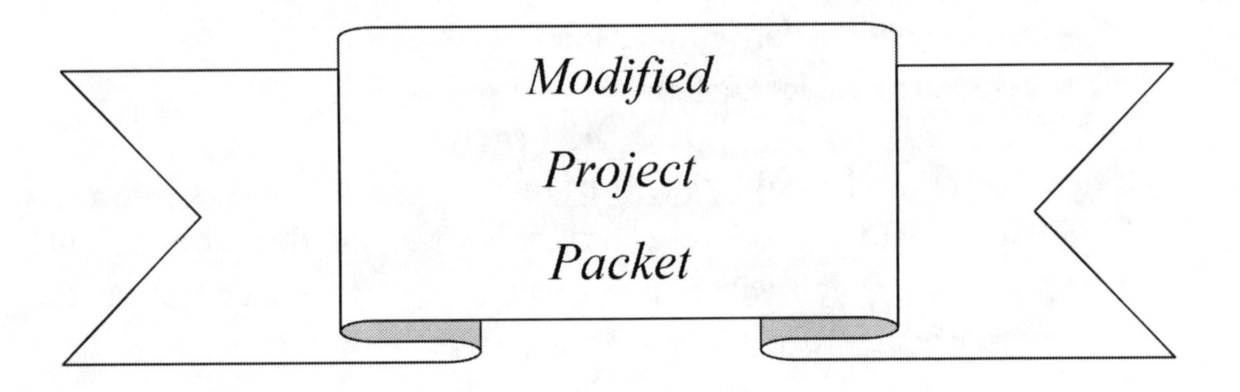

STUDENT NAME: ______________________________

Personal Growth Initiative: Modified Version

Project Requirements

Action: Plan and complete an activity that you have never done before in order to practice the 7 Habits of Highly Effective People.

Required Written Assignments:

- ✓ Project Proposal
- ✓ Supervising Adult Evaluation
- ✓ Student Evaluation Form

Project Poster and Oral Presentation:

You will create a poster that tells the reader about your project. Finally, you will explain your project and poster in an oral presentation to the class. Your poster must include:

- ➢ **A title**
- ➢ **Photos and/or visuals that teach about your project**
- ➢ **A brief description of your project**
- ➢ **Answer to the questions on the Student Evaluation.**

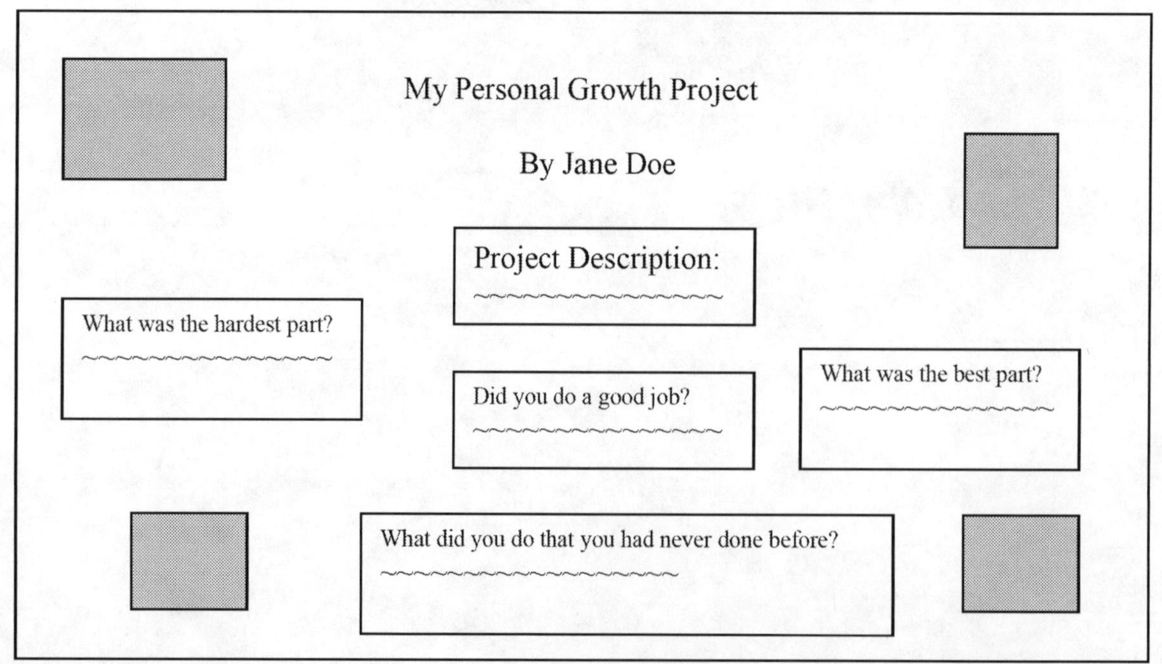

Personal Growth Initiative: Modified Version

Project Proposal

STUDENT NAME: ______________________________ PERIOD: ____ DATE:____

1. **Briefly describe what you plan to do for your project.**

2. **Where will you do this activity?**

3. **When will you do this project?**

4. **Will you do this activity?**
   (circle one) one time many times

5. **Do you need to talk to any adult before starting? If yes, who?**
   (circle one) YES NO

   Who: ____________________

I have read over the project packet, reviewed the completed proposal form, and agree to be a consultant and facilitate my child's project as described above, but I do understand that he/she is responsible to organize and implement this project as much as possible on his/her own.

Signed: ________________________________ Date: ________

Personal Growth Initiative: Modified Version

Student Evaluation

STUDENT NAME: ______________________________ PERIOD: ____ DATE:____

1. **Did you do a good job? Why or why not?**

2. **What was the hardest part?**

3. **What was the best part?**

4. **What did you do that you never had done before?**

STUDENT NAME: ______________________________ PERIOD: ____ DATE:____

Personal Growth Initiative

Supervising Adult Evaluation

1. Did you enjoy your involvement in this activity? Why or Why not?

2. Do you feel the student met his/her overall project goal? Why or Why not?

3. Any suggestions for the student on how his/her project could have been more successful?

4. Can you name any personal attributes or demonstrated behaviors that lead to his/her success?

Thank you for your time and effort in making this project possible! Please sign below to verify the completion of this project evaluation.

Signature: ______________________________ ***Print Name:*** ____________________

Chapter 6: Project Ideas

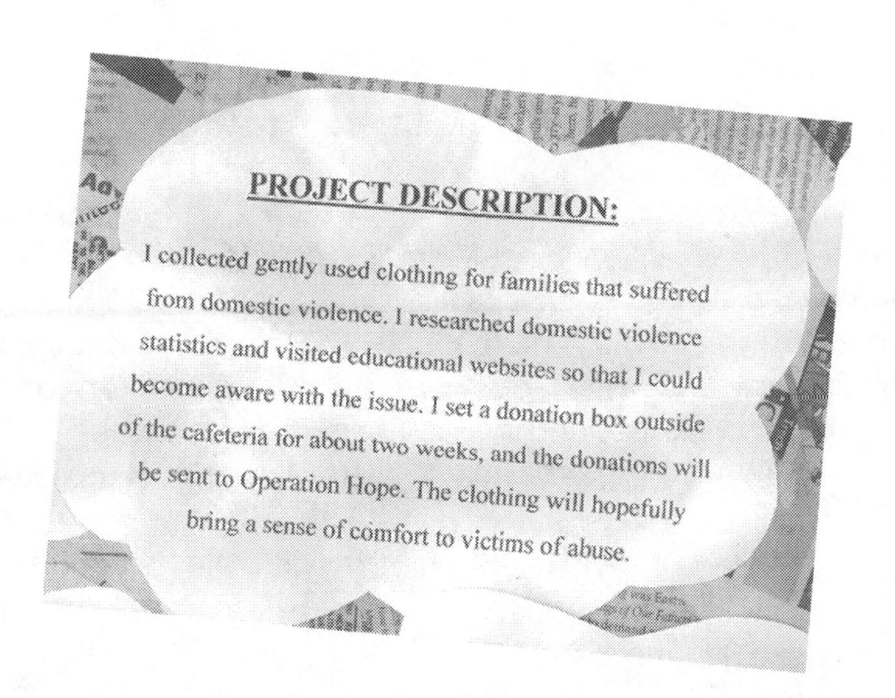

I hesitated on whether or not to include previous students' project ideas in this book because one of the key elements, as you know by now, of a P.G.I. is for the participant to choose their activity based upon their own values and concerns and I feared that these lists might inhibit that process. I would hope you would read this list over so you can get a feel for the incredible possibilities that exist for experiences and to see that the activity choices are pretty boundless because that is true of our students' imaginations.

This list can also serve as a tool to give a basic idea to your students before they start about possible types of activities that can fit into this framework. I usually show former students posters and describe five or so previous project activities to demonstrate the range of simple to complex as well as to show the various different themes (self-improvement, community service, personal connections with family and friends, or acts of kindness). I do also highlight unique opportunities that might exist because of the time of year or season. For instance in the fall ideas around back to school, leaves and planting or Thanksgiving that might trigger an idea for someone, in the winter you have many holidays, cold weather and snow and in the spring there are holidays, gardening and the ability to enjoy the outdoors. Also, there may be something special in your community that you could highlight link to help them become inspired. In our town, each spring a Relay for Life Cancer fundraising marathon is held.

So, for now you can refer to this list, but next time you can use posters and ideas from your own students.

Actual F.W.M.S. Student Projects

- Stocked shelves with donated food at the local food pantry
- Worked at a local farm to earn money and knowledge to buy materials needed for me to grow my own crop of pumpkins.
- Helped neighbor by raking and bagging leaves.
- Helped younger sister's soccer coach with the team practices.
- Helped take care and exercise a horse of a girl with cancer.
- Made a dinner for his nanny who was recovering from surgery.
- Played flute along with a cellist friend for residents at a local nursing home.
- Ran a donation driven drive to help the local wetlands. Picked up trash on a local beach and earned donations based upon how many bags were filled.
- Read and played with young children so their parents could attend temple services.
- Helped friend improve baseball skills, especially batting.
- Kept an elderly neighbor company and helped her get around house.
- Baked holiday desserts to bright spirits of a friend in a nursing home.
- Played clarinet for Alzheimer patients at local convalescent home.
- Read and record easy books in English for use with local elementary ESL students.
- Make and donate quilted blankets to a neo-natal nursery
- Created "name banners" for display outside teacher classrooms.
- Collected lunch trays from teachers' rooms and returned them to the cafeteria.
- Formed a group to sing carols around neighborhood and hand out candy canes.
- Cleaned, stuffed bulletins and set up for church services.
- Made tissue paper flowers and gave them to the elderly at a nursing home.
- Helped staff feed and care for animals at a veterinary hospital.

- Tutor students and assist teacher of religious school classes.
- Collected old cell phones and donated them to a center for battered women and families.
- Help grandfather with chores around the house and yard while he is recovering from surgery.
- Collected recyclable cans for cash used to buy animal treats and supplies for a local animal shelter.
- Offered free babysitting in exchange for donated items needed by the victims of Hurricane Katrina and Rita.
- Planned and supervised his little brother's birthday party.
- Gathered younger kids in the neighborhood for a "science day" and taught about science and did experiments.
- Made breakfast for homeroom classmates and teacher.
- Made posters to raise the visibility of the Salvation Army and Goodwill in our town and show how easy it is to donate to them.
- Taught two younger cousins how to ice skate.
- Made goodie bags and paper flowers for senior citizens for Valentine's Day and St. Patrick's Day.
- Babysat cousins' puppies to prove to parents and herself that she was responsible enough to get a puppy of her own.
- Ran a collection of stuffed animals at two local elementary schools that were sent to poor children in India.
- Collected bottles and can to redeem for cash to help cover the shortage of funds for community outreach program.
- Collected unwanted carpet squares from retail stores to donate to the animal human society for use in cages.
- Organized and held a New Year's Eve party for friends.
- Arranged an in-class party for health classmates to celebrate finishing their research project.
- Mowed lawns for cash that was donated to local homeless shelter.
- Made flashcards and selected easy reader books to use to help sibling with reading skills.
- Sold lollipops to friends and classmates and a chance to win a gift certificate to an ice cream shop to raise

money for foster homes in the area.

- Held a bake sale of personally made items outside of local supermarket and donated the money to the Connecticut Humane Society.
- Sold jewelry made by the Masai tribe from Africa and sent the proceeds back to help the girls attend boarding schools.
- Collect school supplies from neighbors to donate to needy Afghan children.
- Created and sold origami jewelry to donate the profits to cancer research.
- Read a book and did a complimentary activity with an elementary class.
- Read one book to younger sister everyday for four weeks.
- Eliminate chips and cookies from diet for three weeks.
- Helped parents have a relaxing day by doing all needed chores and caring for pets.
- Cared for family hamster, fed it and cleaned cage on a regular basis.
- On Mothers' Day made mother breakfast and did some of her chores.
- Created and supervised a "get in shape" plan for his mother to improve exercise and diet habits.
- Spent Saturdays keeping company with grandmother.
- Washed mother's and father's cars.
- Take nightly walks with parents after having cleaned up litter on their usual route.
- Created a DVD presentation of the family's summer vacation photos and video.
- Taught mother more advanced computer skills.
- Prepared and served an authentic Asian dinner and dessert for family to celebrate their heritage.
- Made flashcards to teach father key Spanish words before a business trip to Spain.
- Earned money by doing chores (learned how to do the dishes and laundry) around his house to donate to a Tsunami relief charity.
- Organized the family' annual vacation; including researching plans and making reservations.
- Volunteered as an assistant coach for the Special Olympic team from Fairfield

- Taught a friend street hockey skills; slapshot, wristshot, snapshot and puck handle.
- Hold a tag sale of items I had helped clean out of our family's attic and basement.
- Organized a group of students from my dance class to perform at a nursing home.
- Collected slightly used athletic equipment and donated it to a local Boys and Girls Club.
- Knit twenty four newborn hats and donated them to Save the Children.
- Presented a series of activities at the public library to raise awareness about food allergies; read a book, handed out brochures and offered allergy free bake goods.
- Volunteered in an inner city after school program twice a week for four weeks. Helped with homework, did crafts and sports.
- Volunteered at the local Audubon Society on weekends. Collected Coca Cola products bottle caps at two grocery stores, an elementary school and our school earning points
- toward funds being sent to the troops in Iraq.
- Helped for four weekends take care of horses and did other stable chores to help the Pegagus Theraputic Riding Program.
- Cooked and served a meal at the local soup kitchen and made treat bags with uplifting messages attached.
- Read the book The Notebook over several visits to a patient at a convalescent home.
- Taught a Brownie troop how to bake a cake and donated it to an inner city after school program.
- Raised awareness about domestic violence with informative posters and collected items needed by the local women's and family center.
- Committed to an exercise routine of running, sit ups and pushups for three weeks to improve my fitness test scores.
- Baked birthday cakes for the children involved in a local Boys and Girls club after school program.
- Taught a math lesson to a fourth grade class.

- Baked cookies with my sisters and gave them to 90 year old neighbor.
- Took a seminar on the exhibits at the Discovery Museum to become a volunteer tour guide.
- At Open House night at the school, held a bake sale and donated the proceeds to the American Cancer Society.
- Created an electric matching board game about Titanic trivia and played it with a 4th grade class after having read them a book about the Titanic.
- Collected local youth sport team jerseys that athletes had outgrown and made them available to those who can not afford to buy new ones.
- Raised fund by selling water bottles at local youth sport sites to donate to a fund that helps families of people awaiting heart transplants.
- Created a webpage for the local animal shelter and posted pictures of the animals needing to be adopted.
- Collected 2500 slightly used books from six elementary schools and organized a book fair for less advantaged kids to keep and have in their classroom libraries.
- Volunteered two days a week at local library in the children's section helping visitors and cataloguing books.
- Solicited from the Scholastic Book company and received over 200 books to donate to the pediatric unit of a local hospital.
- Taught younger neighbors about the flute, played some songs and let them try the instrument.
- Distributed political pamphlets to help a candidate who was running for president.
- Taught sister about scrapbooking while working on a joint scrapbook project.
- Organized a family fun night, chose games, a video and arranged for refreshments.
- Planned and spent a special day with cousin who has cerebral palsy.
- Collected formerly used boys and girls scout uniforms to be donated for those who cannot afford to purchase new ones.

- Organized a bake sale to raise funds for a scholarship fund in honor of a friend's father.
- Created Halloween gift bags for diabetic pediatric patients in an area hospital.
- Weeded an area and planted new plants in Grandparents yard.
- Organized a car wash to raise money for a fund for a local child needing Leukemia treatments.
- Recorded 5 books on tape and donated them to an organization for the blind.
- Organized a surprise birthday part for a friend.
- Wrote and submitted a story about a family friend whose early life was an example in courage during his struggle with Leukemia and many surgeries.
- Gave younger sibling some basic drum lessons
- Lead a sibling's Boy Scoot troop in a collection of magazines and books and composed cards of thanks to soldiers stationed on a medical ship in Iraq.
- Changed light bulbs all over house to energy efficient ones and created a recycling collection system for family to use.
- Organized and played in a quartet benefit concert raising money for the music department in a neighboring community.
- Spend two days working at a Habit for Humanity site where they were building a house in a near by town.
- Hosted a "Green Tea Party". Served green tea and taught peers how teens can conserve energy and help reduce global warming.
- Created a poster about the handling and care of pets; such as hamsters, gerbils and guinea pigs and used it to teach first grade students.
- Cleaned off personal desk at home and created a plan to be more organized and effective with homework.
- Ordered UNICEF boxes and distributed them to friends to collect donations for a good cause while trick or treating

Part Three: Alternative Approaches

Where the Personal Growth Initiative at F.W.M.S. has successfully used the 7 Habits of Highly Effective People as the framework to define and assess the personal growth journey of its participants, it may not suit your needs and wants. We meet our seventh grade health students every day for a marking period. Our P.G.I. framework at F.W.M.S. utilizes approximately three class periods of instruction to get the students up and running and then requires several days for the sharing of the posters at the end of the term. You may not have the ability to allot this amount of class time. Here again, one of the great values of a P.G.I. is how adaptable it can be and as long as the design of the program addresses the key elements; personal growth being the focus, being student driven and the acquiring of personal skills and knowledge you can adapt or use only parts of our framework to better suit your and your students' needs. But you also may imagine one of your own or find one of the upcoming approaches that will fit better into your schedule and time parameters and/or compliment existing curricula.

When I set out to write this book I had only planned to outline the framework we use at F.W.M.S. as I did in Part Two but while I was studying for the three teaching tools H.E.A.P., Choice Theory and Habits of Mind it became apparent to me that these theories and philosophies could be supported by P.G.I. and in turn could be used as frameworks to define and assess such a project. For whatever reason, you may find that one of the three alternative methods I'll outline in this chapter may better fit your personality or program needs. As long as the key elements of a P.G.I are at the heart of your program it will be worthwhile and meaningful. So, keep in mind that ...

> *Personal Growth Initiatives* are structured programs were personal growth is the focus. The design of the experience is student driven and requires the acquisition of personal skills and knowledge.

For each alternative method I give information about the educational theories behind them, describe the focus of the framework and what the project would look like. And though I have never implemented any of these approaches I do believe them to be viable frameworks for a Personal Growth Initiative. Where some of the materials I use with the Seven Habits Framework could be used to enhance these frameworks, I have also created and included worksheets, handouts, rubrics and evaluation sheets specific to each framework.

Chapter 7: National Health Education Standards and H.E.A.P.

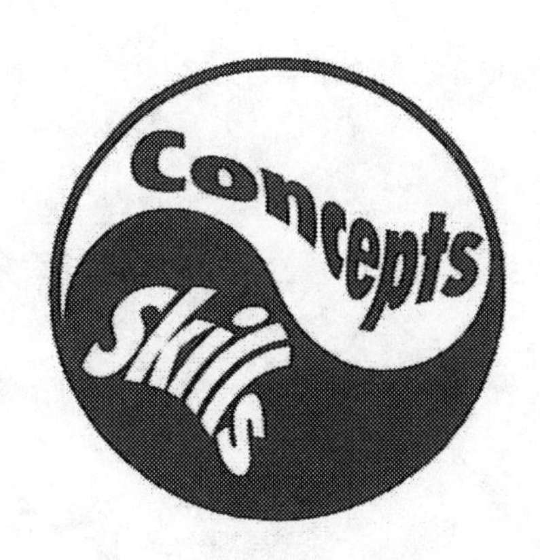

Recently, the middle school and high school Health Education curricula in my town have been revised and are based upon the National Health Education Standards and H.E.A.P. and all the health educators in town have been trained to use HEAP materials. H.E.A.P. stands for Health Education Assessment Project which is a framework of support for instruction and assessment utilizing the seven National Health Education Standards. It became evident to me while working on the curriculum revisions that our P.G.I. addressed each and every one of the seven national standards and is aligned with the H.E.A.P. framework because it has both skill and concept based assessments. It is remarkable that this one project and assessments can satisfy so many curriculum objectives! In that respect, that is why we feel that the class time spent on our P.G.I. is well justified. As I stated earlier, in Chapter 8, the national standards can be used to help justify a Personal Growth Initiative but as I hope to demonstrate the National Health Education Standards and related H.E.A.P. materials could also be an effective alternative approach; driving force and assessment tool for a P.G.I.

THE NATIONAL HEALTH EDUCATION STANDARDS

1. **Core Concepts:** Students will comprehend concepts related to health promotion and disease prevention to enhance health.
2. **Accessing Information:** Students will demonstrate the ability to access valid information and products and services to enhance health.
3. **Analyzing Influences:** Students will analyze the influence of peers, culture, media, technology and other factors on health behaviors.
4. **Self-Management:**
5. **Interpersonal Communications:** Students will demonstrate the ability to use interpersonal communication skills to enhance health and avoid or reduce health risks.
6. **Decision Making & Goal Setting:** Students will demonstrate the ability to use decision-making skills to enhance health. Students will demonstrate the ability to use goal-setting skills to enhance health.
7. **Advocacy:** Students will demonstrate the ability to practice health-enhancing behaviors and avoid or reduce health risks.

WHAT IS H.E.A.P.?

In the hopes of producing health literate students, The Council of Chief State School Officers (CCSSO) and The State Collaborative on Assessment and Student Standards (SCASS) created H.E.A.P. H.E.A.P. stands for Health Education Assessment Project which is a framework of support for instruction and assessment utilizing the seven National Health Education Standards. A Personal Growth Initiative could be an effective instructional tool to foster these traits through practice and assessment. HEAP is founded on the promotion of two dimensions: concepts and skills. Where I will provide a general overview here on the materials and terms I suggest that supervisors choosing this as their approach to a P.G.I. should pursue training with the H.E.A.P. framework and materials.

WHAT WOULD IT LOOK LIKE?

Students could begin their journey of personal growth with learning the definition of Health Literacy. In the report *Healthy People 2010,* the U.S. Department of Health and Human Services included a definition of Health literacy as: "The degree to which individuals have the capacity to obtain, process, and understand basic health information and services needed to make appropriate health decisions".

CCSSO and SCASS have defined a Health Literate people to be a person who:

- " can think through and make healthy choices in solving their own problem"
- "are responsible and make choices that benefit themselves and others"
- "are in charge of their own learning"
- "can use communication skills in clear and respectful ways"

A "student friendly" definition I found in a book titled Totally Awesome Health (by Linda Meeks and Philip Heits) is:

A Health Literate person is a person who is skilled in:

(1) effective communication

(2) self-directed learning

(3) critical thinking

(4) responsible citizenship

Next, students would need to be introduced to the seven National Health Standards; Core Concepts, Accessing Information, Self-Management, Analyzing Influences, Interpersonal Communications, Decision Making & Goal Setting and Advocacy. For your reference, the rationale for each standard and performance indicators from kindergarten through the twelfth grade can be found at www.aahperd.org/aahe/pdf_files/standards.pdf. I have compiled on the following pages display boards that can be used to teach the standards and performance assessment applications for each of the National Health Standards specifically in a P.G.I. These pages can also be made into handouts for students to help with their self-evaluate at the conclusion of their activities.

Now, the students have the needed background knowledge to begin. Students will be instructed to initiate, organize and implement an activity using the seven National Health Standards as their guide and assess the personal growth achieved.

The procedural forms showed earlier; the inventories, the proposal, and evaluation forms that can be found in Chapter 8 could still be used. The final assessments can still take the form of a poster and oral presentation. The poster write-ups would need to address the seven Health Standards and speak to their ability to utilize the prescribed concepts and skills. As H.E.A.P. is designed to be a performance assessment it is equipped with a scoring rubric. It is designed on a four point scale (four to one) with four being the highest score possible and it clearly differentiates levels of performance. These rubrics should be discussed, distributed and displayed.

CCSSO-SCASS Health Education Scoring Rubric

CONCEPTS

4: The response is complex, accurate and comprehensive, showing breadth and depth of information; relationships are described and conclusions drawn.

3: The response identifies relationships between two or more health concepts; there is some breadth of information, although there may be minor inaccuracies.

2: The response presents some accurate information about the relationships between health concepts, but the response is incomplete and there are some inaccuracies.

1: The response addresses the assigned task, but provides little or no accurate information about the relationships between health concepts.

SKILLS

4: The response shows evidence of the ability to apply health skills; the response is complete and shows proficiency in the skill.

3: The response shows evidence of the ability to apply health skills; the response is mostly complete, but may not be fully proficient.

2: The response shows some evidence of the ability to apply health skills. The response may have inaccuracies or be incomplete.

1: The response shows little or no evidence of the ability to apply health skills.

*Taken from HEAP framework manual: CCSSO-SCAS. Health Education Assessment Framework._2003. Print

On the following pages is a sample rubric I developed for a Personal Growth Initiative based on the H.E.A.P. vocabulary, concepts and performance rubrics and handouts outlining the National Health Education standards and each one's connection to such a project. Though these pages look like the ones I offered to be used to justify a P.G.I. they are not, these are intended to be used with the students and are worded as learning objectives.

Personal Growth Initiative Grading Sheet: H.E.A.P.

STUDENT NAME: ______________________ PERIOD:____ DATE:___

ORAL PRESENTATION

RUBRIC AND POINT EARNINGS

Area	AWESOME	ACCEPTABLE	MINIMAL	UNACCEPTABLE
Content description	Clearly overviewed project, reason for choosing it, project's goal and personal growth	Described project and goal	Some explanation of project	Little to no project
Delivery	Clear voice, loud, and pleasant Showed confidence, comfort and high degree of understanding. and preparation	Adequate voice tone and volume Appeared confident and prepared.	Low voice quality and showed little confidence and effort.	Voice tone or volume took away from delivery. Showed little to no evidence of preparation
	(25-30 points)	(15-25 points)	(5-15 points)	(0-5points)

ORAL PRESENTATION = _____ POINTS

VISUAL PRESENTATION= _____ POINTS

TOTAL POINTS= _____

FINAL GRADE=

VISUAL PRESENTATION (pg.2)
POSTER RUBRIC AND POINT EARNINGS

Area	AWESOME	ACCEPTABLE	MINIMAL	UNACCEPTABLE
Performance Assessment	Earned mostly 4s on the concept and skill ratings (29-32 points)	Earned mostly 3s on the concept and skill ratings (23-28 points)	Earned mostly 2s on the concept and skill ratings (15-22 points)	Earned mostly 1s on the concept and skill ratings (0-14 points)
Overall Content	Well-written captions that illustrate and inform about a meaningful project and how it fostered Health Literacy. (20-23 points)	Captions that inform viewer about the project, and it's impact on Health Literacy. (16-19 points)	Captions inform minimally or are incomplete about (10-15 points)	Text is non-existent, incomplete, inaccurate, or fail to inform (0-9 points)
Design	Layout contains appropriate photos or visuals that are easily read, logical and neat. (4-5 points)	Layout contains photos, is mostly neat, fairly logical and easy to understand . (3-4 points)	Somewhat disorganized; and hard to understand. (2-3 points)	Disorganized; appears unplanned and done hastily. (1-2 points)
Visual	Visuals capture viewer's attention and interest and are effective. (4-5 points)	Good use of color and eye-catching elements (3-4 points)	Some good ideas but something detracts from the message. (2-3 points)	Color, photos or graphic details minimal or poorly done. (1-2 points)
Creativity	Uses ideas, and/or design elements that are unexpected or original. (4-5 points)	Contains some unique or imaginative ideas. (3-4 points)	Shows some attempts at creativity (2-3 points)	Little or no evidence of creativity. (1-2 points)

CORE CONCEPTS

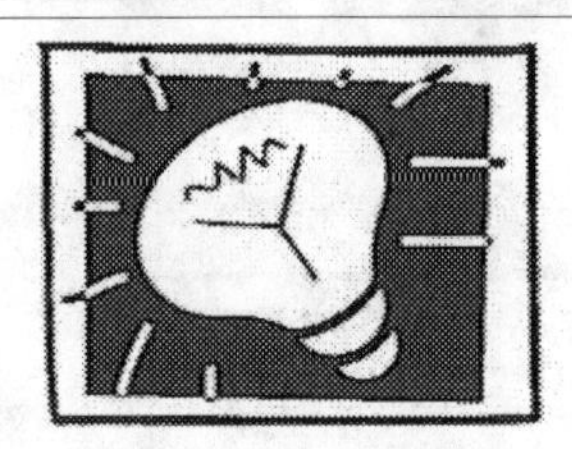

HEALTH EDUCATION STANDARD 1: Students will comprehend concepts related to health promotion and disease prevention.

You will/can...

1. Identify the concepts utilized to promote health and/or prevent unhealthy behaviors.

2. Show relationships among ideas and concepts.

3. Make conclusions about accuracy of information.

ACCESSING INFORMATION

HEALTH EDUCATION STANDARD 2:
Students will demonstrate the ability to access valid health information and health-promoting products and services.

You will/can...

1. Identify sources of information and resources.

2. Analyze how sources impact project's success.

SELF MANAGEMENT

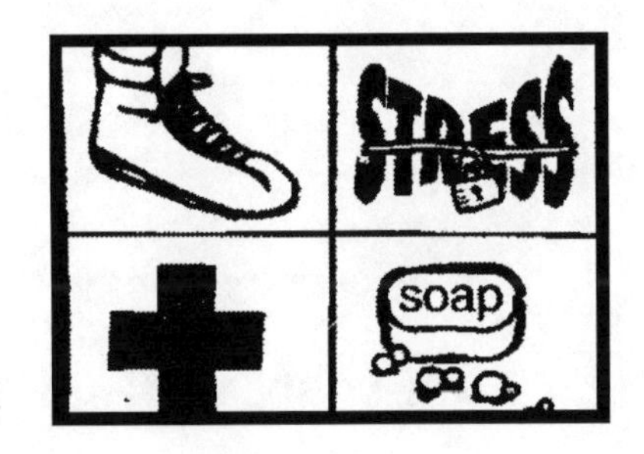

HEALTH EDUCATION STANDARD 3:
Students will demonstrate the ability to practice health enhancing behaviors and reduce health risks

You will/can...

1. Demonstrate habits that contribute to health.

2. Explain how steps taken have improved health.

ANALYZING INFLUENCES

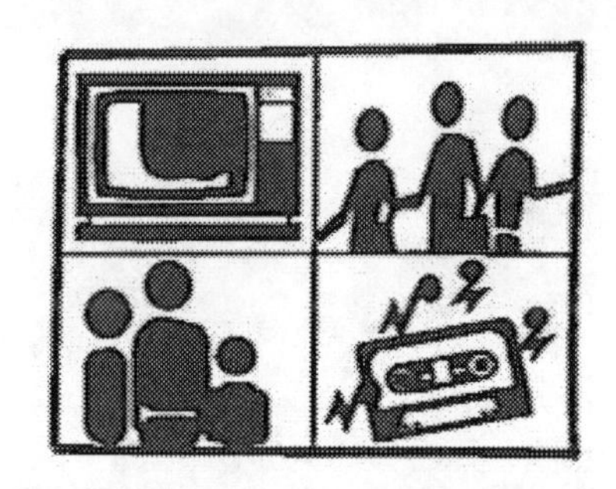

HEALTH EDUCATION STANDARD 4:
Students will analyze the influence of culture, media, technology, and other facts on health.

You will/can...

1. Identify internal and external influences that contributed to project's success.

2. Explain about influences that may affect future health behaviors.

INTERPERSONAL COMMUNICATION

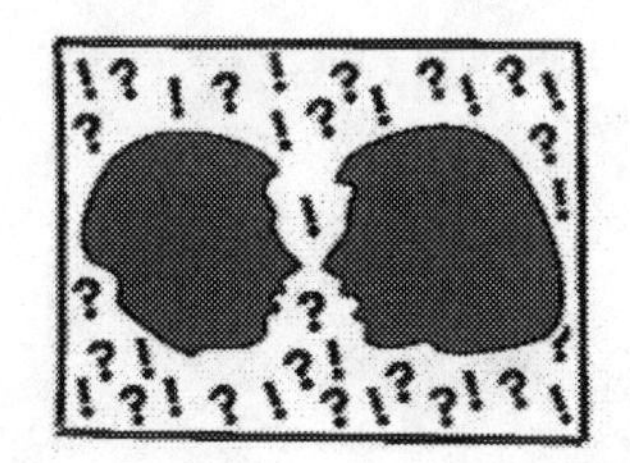

HEALTH EDUCATION STANDARD 5:
Students will demonstrate the ability to use interpersonal comunication skills to enhance health.

You will/can...

1. Demonstrate ability to actively listen for content and meaning.

2. Demonstrate ability to clearly express ideas and needs.

3. Analyze how communication skills improved performance.

DECISION MAKING

HEALTH EDUCATION STANDARD 6:
Students will demonstrate the ability to use goal-setting and decision making skills to enhance health.

You will/can...

1. Identify options and possibilities that were considered.

2. Identify the decisions made.

3. Evaluate how the decisions impacted the outcome.

GOAL SETTING

HEALTH EDUCATION STANDARD 6: Students will demonstrate the ability to use goal-setting and decision making skills to enhance health.

You will/can...

1. Create goal(s).

2. Design a plan to meet goal(s).

3. Demonstrate how to evaluate and adjust plan if needed.

ADVOCACY

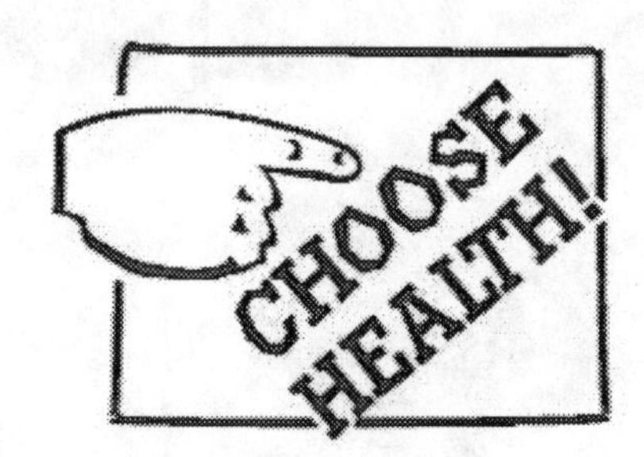

HEALTH EDUCATION STANDARD 7: Students will demonstrate the ability to advocate for personal, family and community health.

You will/can...

1. Create a meaningful goal based on values and concerns.

2. Reflect upon personal growth and impact on others.

3. Share goals and project.

Chapter 8: Control Theory and Responsibility Training

CONTROL THEORY

During my sixth year degree coursework I took an online course offered by Quality Education Programs, Inc. titled Teaching Students Responsible Behavior. The coursework uses teaching from William Glasser, M.D. and utilizes his Control Theory and Responsibility Training model. Quite smugly as I delved into these philosophies and practices I realized how well our P.G.I. addresses and support them.

WHAT IS CONTROL THEORY?

Control Theory which was once called Choice Theory, teaches that the brain gives everyone the self-directing capability that is required to fulfill life needs. These teachings help students understand they choose their own behaviors and to help them gain control over their lives.

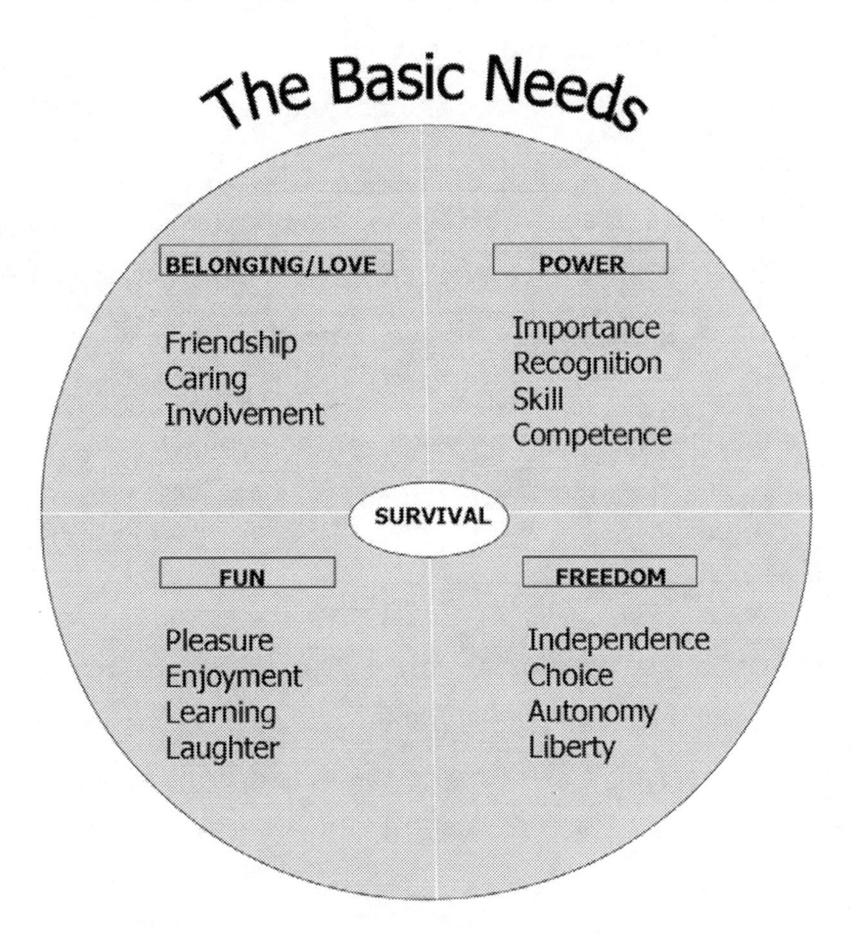

People are driven by six basic needs. All of our choices and behaviors are based upon the urgency for survival, power, love, belonging, freedom and fun. Decisions are based upon how what is happening in “the now” matches with a person’s vision of a “quality world” or a “good life”. The brain is a “good life” control center that designs and directs behavior based upon emotions and sensory information.

Students who study Control Theory are taught that emotions are life’s “natural evaluation system”. They feel glad when they choose behaviors that fulfill one or more of their needs; mad when they don’t get what they want; sad when they lose something special and afraid when they do not feel safe or do not know how to make things better. As they learn to understand their own need based behaviors they can be taught to satisfy their needs in a responsible and healthful way.

The main axioms of Control Theory are:

- All behavior is need and goal driven.
- All behavior, whether good or bad, is an attempt to satisfy those needs
- All behaviors are made of four components: acting, thinking, feeling and physiology. We only have direct control over the acting and thinking components. We can only control our feeling and physiology through how we choose to act and think.
- The only person whose behavior we can control is our own.

WHAT WOULD IT LOOK LIKE?

I envision using Control Theory as a P.G.I. alternative could be less time and work intensive because teaching the Control Theory is less complex than the first two approaches. A class period could be spent on introducing the concepts and having them investigate ways that they meet these basic needs currently.

Examining the basic needs; there are physical and psychological needs. Our physical needs involve "surviving". This need necessitates that we behave in ways that produce food, shelter and safety. All other needs are psychological. "Belonging" is the need that requires that we be connected to our world; to be with people who know and care about us and to be accepted and appreciated. The need for "Gaining Power" demands that we learn, gain knowledge and skills. The more we know, the more we can do the more our self-esteem grows. "Having Fun" is the need that mandates that we behave in ways that bring joy and satisfaction into our lives. It results from accomplishments, recreation and entertainment. The need for "Being Free" necessitates us to be in control of our lives; to set goals, to make plans, to choose behaviors, to evaluate results and to decide what to do next. After this material is presented, I would have them complete the chart below with at least three things in their lives or current behaviors that support each basic need. I have done this activity with classes in two different ways; they can fill the box in with pictures or words.

Here is a sample that could be used as a model.

The Four Basic Needs

BELONGING / LOVE	POWER
Having a family Teamwork Having friends Being a part of a club Caring for pets	Doing my best Learning new things Solving problems myself Feeling good about myself Getting acknowledgements
HAVING FUN	**BEING FREE**
Playing Games Winning Laughing Talking to friends Doing things you like	Choose what to do next Make a new friend Plan for the future To be myself!

Student Name: ______________________ Period: ___

The Four Basic Needs

BELONGING / LOVE	POWER
HAVING FUN	**BEING FREE**

At the next class period the project could be explained to the students. This project is a P.G.I. where they will need to initiate, organize and implement an activity that they have never done before and assess which of the basic needs were supported or satisfied during the process. They will need to enlist an adult to act as observer and evaluator. Much of the previous materials could still be used including, the Inventories, proposal form and even the student and adult supervisor evaluation sheets.

The final assessments still could take the form of a poster and oral presentation. The poster write-ups would need to address which decisions, behaviors and results satisfied each of the basic four needs. I believe they could use visuals as well as words to express their thinking. The original rubric might need to be slightly modified but could be used. In addition, you could ask your students to go to a higher level of reflection to compare their "before" and "after" basic need charts. They could share these revelations either during their oral presentations or in a writing piece.

RESPONSIBILITY TRAINING

WHAT IS RESPONSIBILITY TRAINING?

What I have outlined above was what I had originally envisioned as a "quicker hit" type of P.G.I. As I reviewed my materials and work from my course I realized that if I give you some background on Responsibility Training it could be another viable alternative approach for a P.G.I. This approach requires more instructional time and goes in a different direction because it is based upon targeting personal behaviors, tracking and assessing progress.

By definition, Responsibility Training is a life skills learning program and is Control Theory in action. Responsibility Training uses G-PAR as a behavior improvement plan for creating goals from needs, making plans to achieve those goals, taking action to implement the plan, evaluating results. These strategies require that students choose their own behaviors to target an area for personal improvement and reflect upon the results. See, it really is a perfect fit to be included in a P.G.I.

G-PAR STRATEGIES:

1. My Goals: This is how I get what I really want.
2. My Plan: This is how I think about how to get what I really want.
3. My Actions: This is the behavior I choose to carry out my plan.
4. My Results: Through information from my senses (ears, eyes, nose, skin) and my feelings I can determine if I did get what I wanted.

In this approach, after introducing Control Theory and giving your students a chance to apply the basic needs concepts to their own lives (chart activity) I suggest you have a discussion on what is their definition of responsibility? And discuss what is seen as values of being responsible? And in what ways could being responsible meet any of one's basic needs? What does it mean to be irresponsible? What are some consequences to behaving irresponsibly?

> **Responsibility** is literally "the ability to respond", the ability to react to input, the ability to respond to the world around us.

So, what does *Being Responsible* look like? To describe behaviors of a responsible person most people would use synonyms like; careful, conscientious, reliable, mature, stable, sensible, effective, dependable, predictable, trustworthy and hard working. Responsible people tend to be productive, confident, cooperative and happy because they satisfy their basic needs. The obvious basic needs that responsible behavior meets are gaining power and being free. But because healthy people are drawn to surround themselves with responsible people belonging and having fun can often be met too. However, if someone acts irresponsibly it indicates that they do not have the ability to respond and feel that they have no control over making "their now" match their "good life" vision. Irresponsible behaviors include missing deadlines, procrastination, acting in haste, disregarding rules or consequences and blaming others. Irresponsible behavior works against achieving all of one's basic needs.

After this discussion, you could introduce the G-PAR strategies and materials. Students would be asked to complete some personal inventories to aid in the reflection needed to create a meaningful goal. I have included here some materials I created for this purpose as well as tools to aid in the planning, progress reporting and an evaluation sheet for the participant and adult consultant.

Personal Growth Initiative: Responsibility Training

G-PAR Personal Inventory

Student Name: ______________________________ Period: ___

<u>Directions:</u> Complete each section with the requested information after taking time to reflect. Be honest and sincere! You are not going to share this with others so you do not have to impress anyone but you.

- Name three people that you really admire (friends, family, teachers, coaches, etc) and name the qualities about them that you admire.

Name	Qualities You Admire

- Briefly describe the person you would like to be. (personal qualities, reputation, health, appearance, skills, knowledge, future career)

____

____

____

____

- Name three qualities that you would like the people in your life to use to describe you? They do not have to be true of you now.

FAMILY	FRIENDS	TEACHERS

- List three behaviors that are helping you become the person you want to be and explain how you know that it's helping you.

Helping Behaviors	How you know it's helping

- List three behaviors that are blocking you from become the person you want to be and how these behaviors negatively impact what you want.

Blocking Behaviors	Negative Impact

Personal Growth Initiative: Responsibility Training

G-PAR GOAL SHEET

Student Name: ______________________________ Period: ___

Directions: Complete each section with the requested information after taking time to reflect. Be honest and sincere!

- In the basic need charting activity...

  Which basic needs (gaining power, having fun, being free, belonging/love) were the easiest to come up with examples from your life?

  ____

  Which basic needs (gaining power, having fun, being free, belonging/love) were the hardest to come up with examples from your life?

  ____

- Review your Inventory Sheet where you listed three blocking behaviors, which basic needs would you say you are trying to fulfill when you choose each behavior.

Blocking Behaviors:	**Basic Needs (Love, Power, Freedom, Fun**
Blocking Behavior 1	
Blocking Behavior 2	
Blocking Behavior 3	

- **The basic need that I really want to work on improving is ______________.**

I will create a plan to gain personal growth in the area of _____________ so the "real me" will get closer to the vision of myself I want to be. I will seek feedback on my progress from an adult.

Signed: ________________________________ Date: _____

Personal Growth Initiative: Responsibility Training

G-PAR PLAN SHEET

Student Name: ______________________________ Period: ___

Directions: Develop a realistic plan of action toward achieving your goal and a system to track your progress.

1. The basic need that I really want to work on improving is _______________.

2. My adult consultant will be:

_________________________ (name)

_________________________ (relationship)

3. The **behaviors I must stop** are:

Behaviors	When & Where & With Whom

4. The **behaviors I must start** are:

Behaviors	When & Where & With Whom

Personal Growth Initiative: Responsibility Training

G-PAR TRACKING PROGRESS SHEET

Student Name: ______________________________ Period: ___

Directions: Begin by writing in the actual behaviors you are targeting on the top of each column. Reflect weekly upon your P.G.I.; your goal and your action plan. Then put an "x" next to the corresponding number that you feel represents your performance this week for each behavior. The performance rating is on a scale from one to ten. 10 represents one hundred percent of the time you were successful, 5 would represent fifty percent and so on.

Student Name: _ _ _ _ _ _ _ _ _ _ _ _ _ _ _ _ _ _ Date Chart Completed: _ _ _ _ _

PERFORMANCE RATING	BEHAVIORS					
10						
9						
8						
7						
6						
5						
4						
3						
2						
1						
0						

Personal Growth Initiative: Responsibility Training

G-PAR EVALUATION SHEET

Student Name: ______________________________ Period: ___

<u>Directions:</u> Review your pre-project paperwork and reflect upon your planning, actions and the results. Answer the questions below to demonstrate a high degree of reflection and learning.

1. How well did you follow your plan? What evidence supports your claim?

2. Did you get the results that you wanted? How do you know?

3. How did you feel as a result of this project?

4. Which behavior change are you most proud of and why?

5. Were there any results that surprised you? (for example; another need was also met, people's reactions to your changed behavior, your successes or hardships)

6. What is the next step toward improving yourself? Will you keep working on this goal or a new goal?

7. <u>Get feedback from your adult consultant:</u> Share your answers from above with your adult consultant. Then ask him/her following questions, write the answers below and have them sign at the bottom of this page.

   - On a scale of 1-10 how well did the students follow the plan. _____
   - Which behavior change was the most important? Why?
   - Do you have any suggestions to help this student to continue to grow and improve?

Adult Consultant Signature: ______________________________ **Date:** ____

Chapter 9: Habits of Mind

I was introduced to the Habits of Mind through professional development workshops at my school. My school and the two other middle schools in town have established short and long term building wide objectives regarding developing the Habits of Mind in our students. Simply put, the goal is to infuse the curricula and school environments with Habits of Mind concepts and skills. My personal professional goals for the last two years have centered on introducing these terms and concepts into my existing curricula and my involvement on a committee to develop ways to raise awareness and practice of the Habits of Mind in the school community. When I met Bena Kallick, co-creator and author of the Habits of Mind, we spoke about the Personal Growth Initiative at FWMS (of which she was very impressed) and we discussed the real potential of utilizing the Habits of Mind in such a project. I'll begin by offering a brief overview of the sixteen habits, suggest how to teach the habits to your students and offer some thoughts of how I see them being a part of a very productive and meaningful personal growth initiative.

WHAT ARE THE HABITS OF MIND?

After years of study into Intellectual Behaviors, Bena Kallick and Arthur Costa named what they saw as dispositions to effective thinking. These intelligent behaviors are most vital under challenging conditions such as, situations where the explanation or answer to a problem, stimulus, question or task is not immediately known. Therefore, the premise of this educational movement is to have our students develop more than just knowing the right answers, but to also develop how to behave when answers are not immediately apparent.

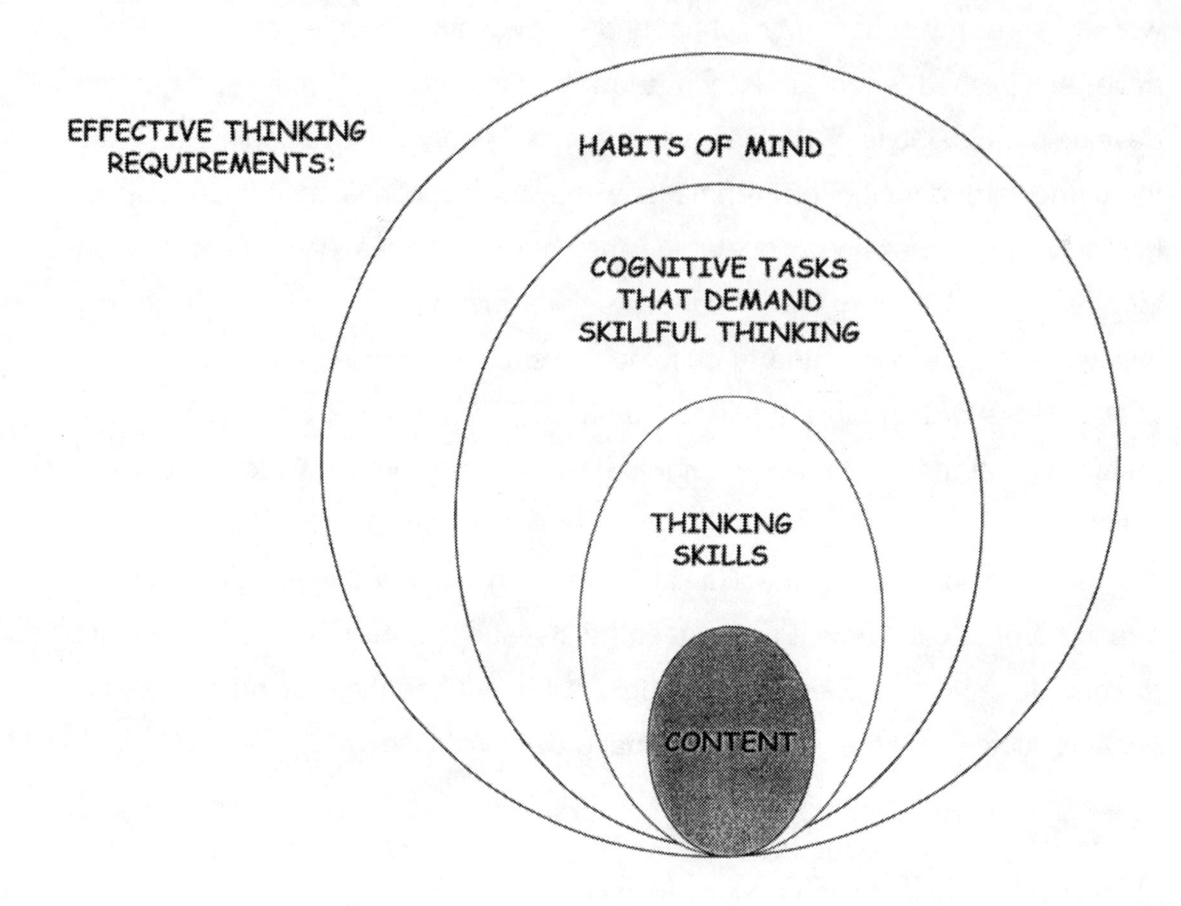

The authors say that these sixteen behaviors that they have identified require discipline of the mind and practice so they will become habits that will lead toward more thoughtful, intelligent actions. I encourage you to read for greater understanding and instructional ideas in the book series titled, Habits of Mind - A Developmental Series which can be found at http://www.habits-of-mind.net The following chart gives a brief definition of each of the habits.

The Habits of Mind

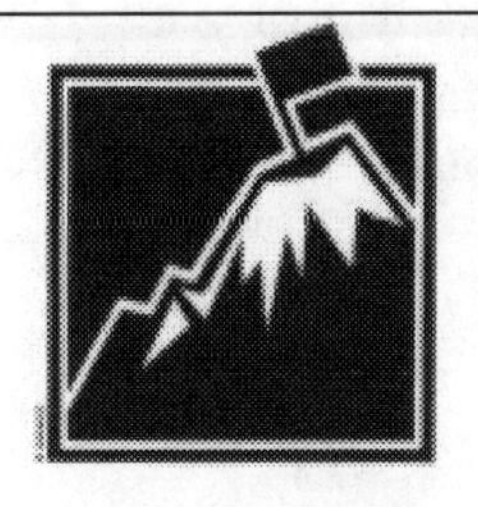	***Persistence*** Stick to it! Persevering in task through to completion; remaining focused. Looking for ways to reach your goal when stuck. Not giving up
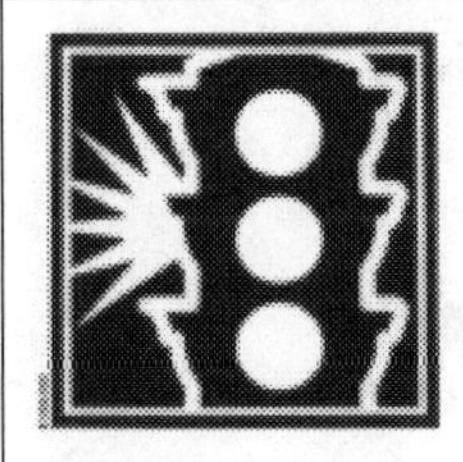	***Managing Impulsivity*** Take your Time! Thinking before acting; remaining calm, thoughtful and deliberative.
	***Listening with Empathy and Understanding*** Understand Others! Devoting mental energy to another person's thoughts and ideas; Make an effort to perceive another's point of view and emotions
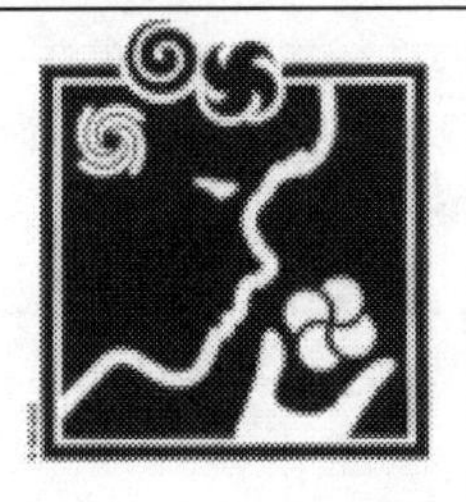	***Thinking Flexibly*** Look at it Another Way! Being able to change perspectives, generate alternatives, consider options

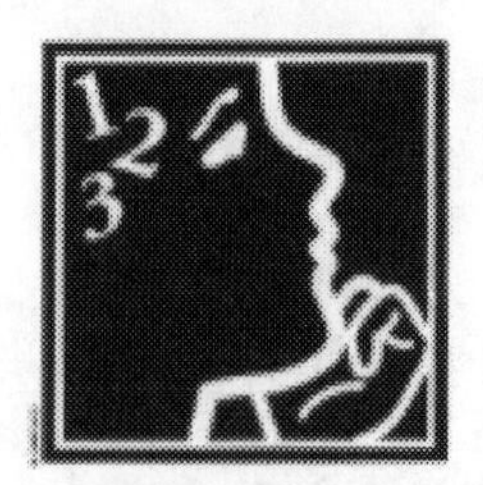	***Thinking about your Thinking : Metacognition*** Know your knowing! Being aware of your own thoughts, strategies, feelings and actions and their effects on others.
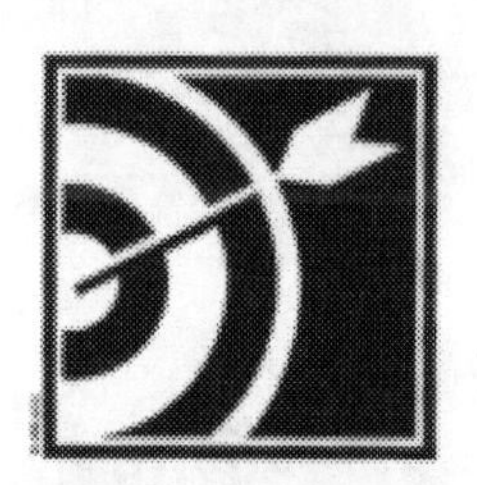	***Striving for Accuracy*** Check it again! Always doing your best. Setting high standards. Checking and finding ways to improve constantly.
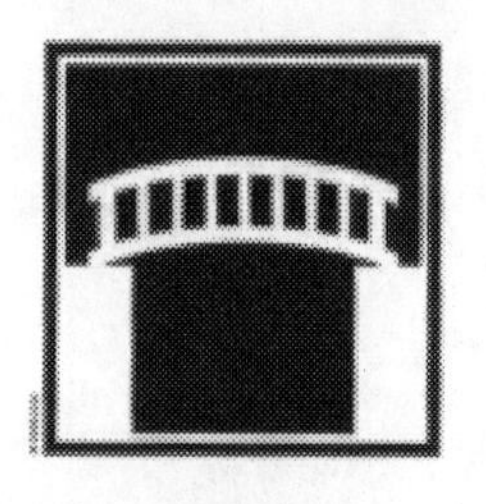	***Applying Past Knowledge*** Use what you Learn! Accessing prior knowledge; transferring knowledge beyond the situation in which it was learned.
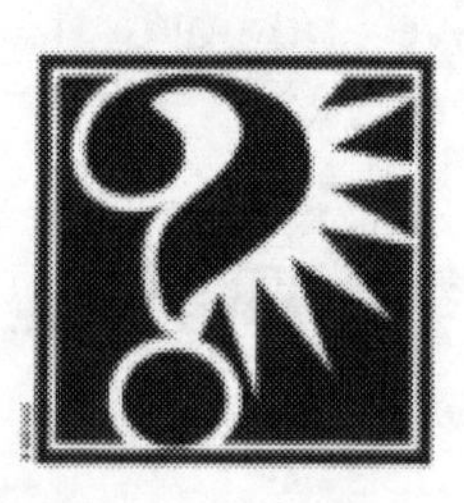	***Questioning and Posing Problems*** How do you know? Having a questioning attitude; knowing what data are needed and developing questioning strategies to produce those data. Finding problems to solve

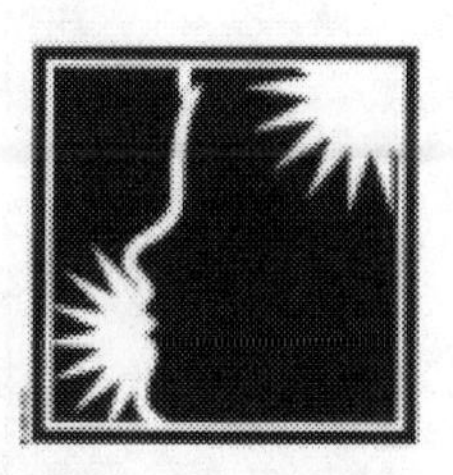	***Thinking and Communicating with Clarity and Precision*** Be clear! Striving for accurate communication in both written and oral form; avoiding over generalizations, distortions, deletions and exaggerations.
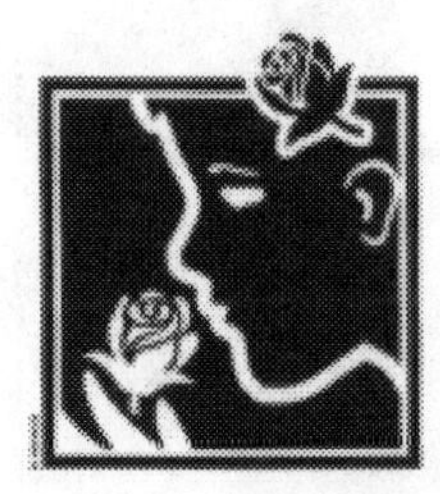	***Gathering Data Through All Senses*** Use your natural pathways! Pay attention to the world around you Gather data through all the senses. taste, touch, smell, hearing and sight
	***Creating, Imagining & Innovating*** Try a different way! Generating new and novel ideas, fluency, originality
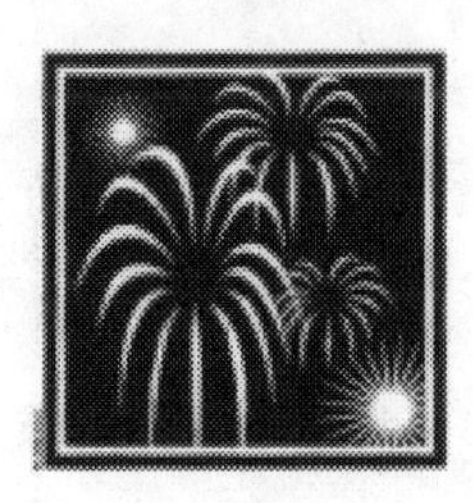	***Responding With Wonderment and Awe*** Have fun figuring it out! Finding the world awesome, mysterious and being intrigued with phenomena and beauty. Being passionate.

	***Taking Responsible Risks*** Venture out! Being adventuresome; living on the edge of one's competence. Try new things constantly.
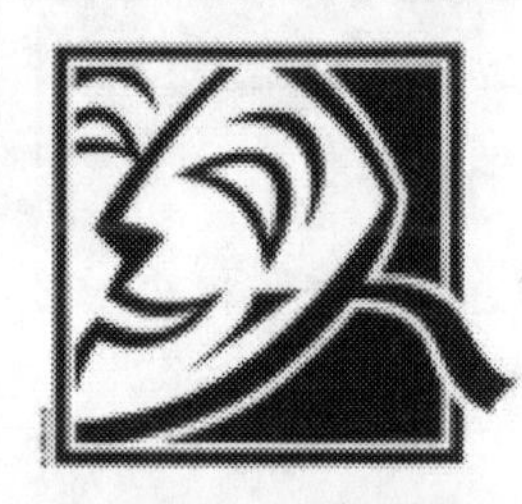	***Finding Humor*** Laugh a little! Finding the whimsical, incongruous and unexpected. Being able to laugh at oneself.
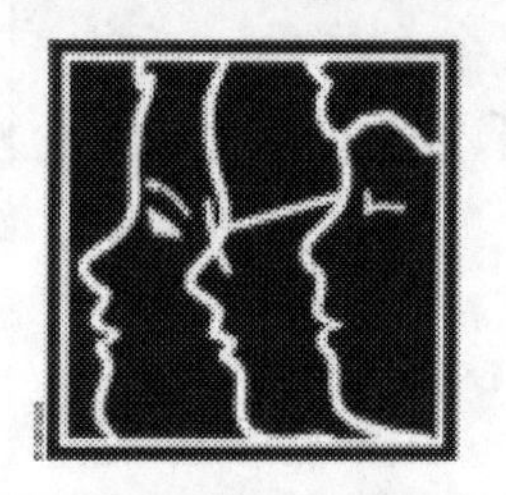	***Thinking Interdependently*** Work together! Being able to work in and learn from others in reciprocal situations. Team work.
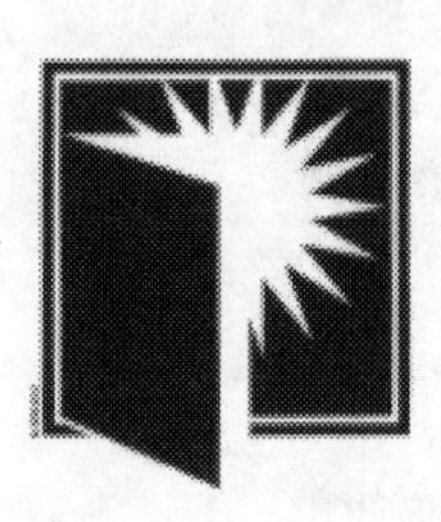	***Remaining Open to Continuous Learning*** Learn from experiences! Having humility and pri when admitting we don't know; resisting complacency.

http://www.habitsofmind.org

TEACHING THE HABITS OF MIND

In my case, my students have been exposed to these concepts in all their classes. They have been introduced to how these behaviors could help them in everyday life, their academic and "art" (art, music, health, computers, family consumer science, and technical education) classes. We have also held assemblies and activities that focused on specific habits. I'm hoping that this might be true for some of you reading this too and if it is the case than this approach would be a terrific match and probably the easiest way for you to incorporate a personal growth initiative with your students. If not, how you go about teaching the sixteen habits would be determined by how much class time you can allocate. I suggest that there are too many habits to spend class time teaching about each habit before starting the P.G.I. You could ask your students to read about each habit outside of class and perform an assessment to demonstrate their understanding before you begin, or you could have them break into pairs or small groups and have them become "experts" on one habit and have each group teach their classmates about their habit.

WHAT WOULD IT LOOK LIKE?

There are various strategies you could use to confirm your students' understanding of the concepts and skills related to the habits. You could ask them to individually or in small groups create "Word Splashes" for some or all of the habits. A Word Splash" is a list of words or phrases that could be considered synonyms or attributes associated with the habit. You could have them personalize their learning by rating how often they practice this habit currently and determine five or so that they most need to work on and describe why. I have created a worksheet that could be used.

The Habits of Mind: Personal Survey

HOW MUCH DO I CURRENTLY PRACTICE THEM?

Directions: Put an "X" in the box that best represents to what degree you think you practice the habit: Never, Seldom, Sometimes, Often or Always. Then respond to the reflection
Now, go back and **circle the five habits** you identify as the most important for you to focus on developing in the near future.

THE HABITS OF MIND	NEVER	SELDOM	SOMETIMES	OFTEN	ALWAYS
Persisting "Sticking to it"					
Thinking and communicating with clarity and precision questions to assess your results. "Being clear when you communicate"					
Managing impulsivity "Take your time"					
Gathering data through all senses "Use all your natural resources"					
Listening with understanding and empathy "Work to understand others"					
Creating, imagining, innovating "Try new and different ways"					
Thinking flexibly "Able to change and consider options"					
Responding with wonderment and awe "Intrigued by things and events"					
Thinking about thinking (Metacognition) "Knowing your own thoughts, feelings and actions"					
Taking responsible risks "Adventurous or willing to try new things"					
Striving for accuracy "Work precisely and for exactness"					
Finding humor "Being able to laugh and see fun in things"					
Questioning and posing problems "Asking questions and wanting to learn more"					
Thinking interdependently "Able to work and learn from others"					
Applying past knowledge to new situations "Able to see connections"					
Remaining open to continuous learning "being open to new things and ideas"					

Which one do you think will be the easiest for you? ______________________

Which one do you think will be the hardest for you? ______________________

You, or your students, could create a matching worksheet or a card game with the names of the habits and descriptions. Other possible strategies include; creating a symbol or logo or create a simile or slogan representing the habits, giving examples of what people would say if they were using that habit or to describe situations when it is important to use the habit. You could also ask them to make it personal and ask them to describe a time when they used this habit or wished they had used this habit in their own lives. Also, as a tool to assess their understanding and reinforce each habit you could have them create mini-posters to be displayed around the room. They could use pictures, words, phrases and quotes to demonstrate their learning or if individuals or groups were assigned to teach their classmates about one specific habit they could use their mini-poster as a visual aid. I have created a mini-poster for the habit of "persistence" which could be used as a sample.

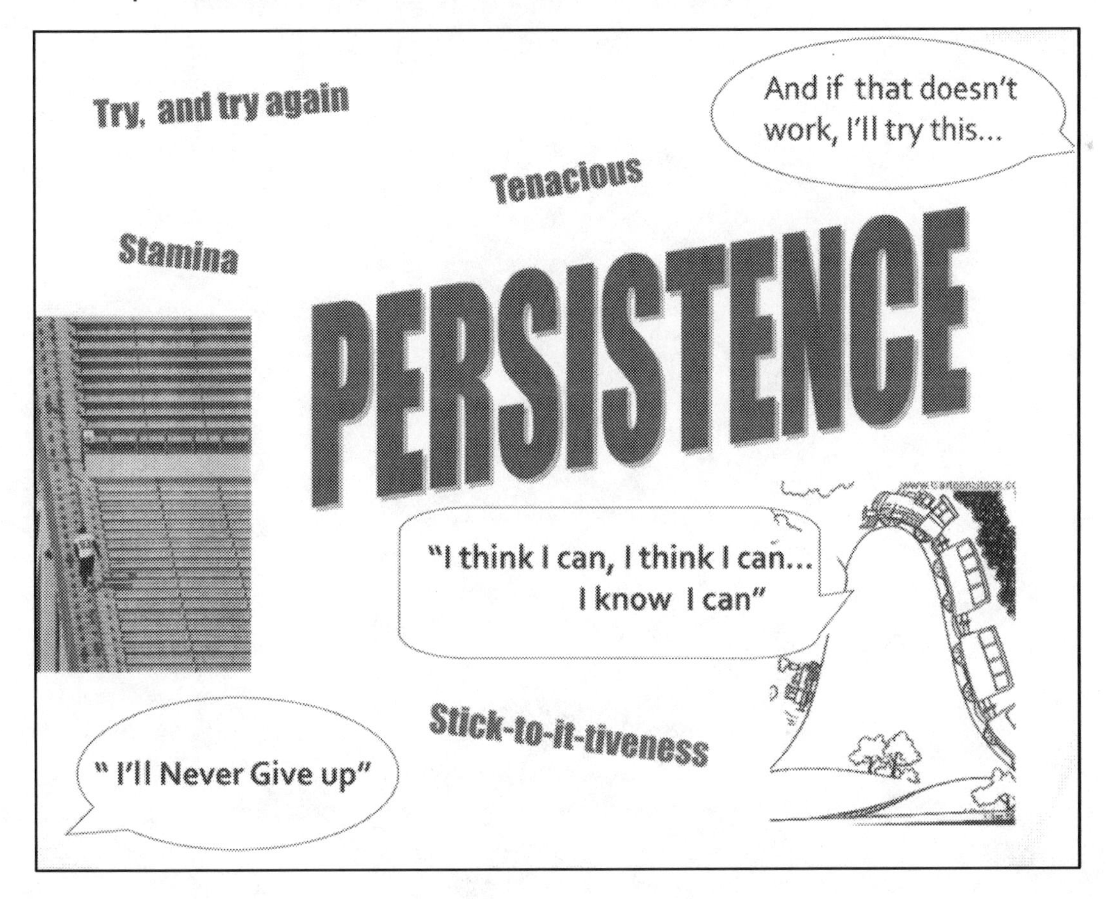

After the students have the needed background knowledge to begin. Students will be instructed to initiate, organize and implement an activity using the Habits of Mind as their guide and tool for assessing their personal growth. You as the supervisor will need to determine the protocol that meets your needs and constraints. I probably would begin with the participant using the information from the Personal Survey results to base the identification of three to five habits to target. Below I have made a sample project proposal/goal sheet as well as student and adult evaluation sheets. The final assessments could still take the form of a poster and oral presentation. The poster write-ups would need to address the Habits of Mind the individual was targeting and speak to their practice of the prescribed concepts and skills. I have added a modified rubric to suit the needs of this approach.

Personal Growth Initiative: Habits of Mind

Project Requirements

Action: Plan and complete an activity that will allow you to practice the Habits of Mind .

Required Written Assignments:

- ✓ Project Proposal/Goal Sheet
- ✓ Supervising Adult Evaluation
- ✓ Student Evaluation Form

Project Poster and Oral Presentation:

You will create a poster that teaches about your project, identifies the Habits of Mind that you were targeting and describes how well you practiced them. Finally, you will explain your project and poster in an oral presentation to the class and demonstrate your understanding of the related terms. Your poster must include:

- **A title**
- **Photos and/or visuals that teach about your project**
- **A brief description of your project**
- **The names of the Habits of Minds you were addressing and a write-up of how well you practiced them.**

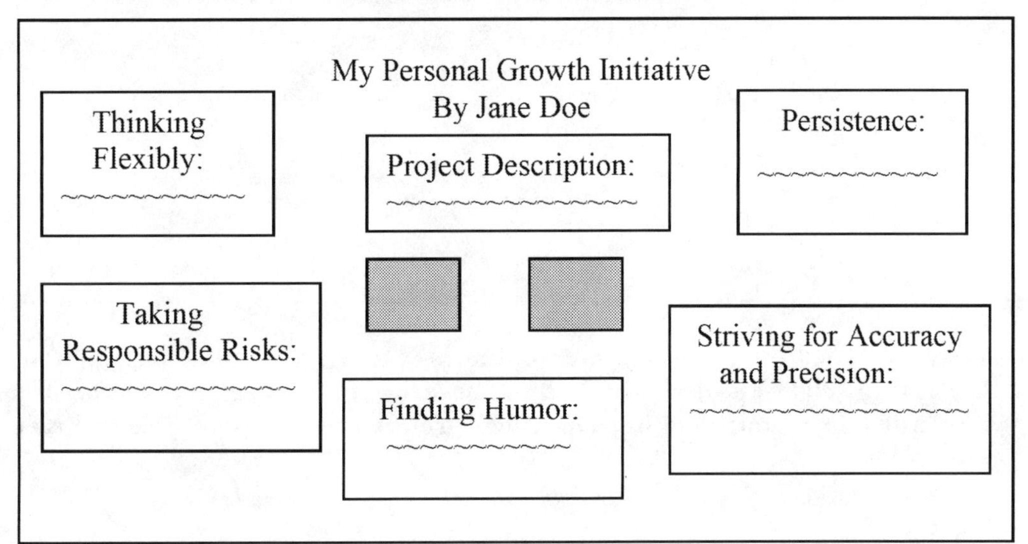

Personal Growth Initiative: Habits of Mind

Proposal/Goal Sheet

Student Name: ________________________________ Period: ____

1. Briefly describe what you hope to do for your project:

2. What aspect of this activity will you be doing for the first time?

3. List below **the Habits of Mind** you plan to mindfully practice during this project and briefly **explain why you have chosen them.**

Habits of Mind	Rationale (Why?)

I have reviewed the completed proposal form, and agree to be a consultant and facilitate my child's project as described above, but I do understand that he/she is responsible to organize and implement this project as much as possible on his/her own.

Signed: ________________________________ **Date:** _______________

Personal Growth Initiative: Habits of Mind

Student Evaluation

STUDENT NAME: ______________________________ DATE: ____

1. Do you feel your project was successful? Circle one:
   YES NO SOMEWHAT

2. Why do you feel it was successful or unsuccessful?

3. Were there any ways you could have been more successful?

4. What behaviors or actions did you do that you had never done before?

5. What personal learning or insights will you carry forward to future situations?

6. Based upon your participation in this activity what behaviors might you…stop doing? continue doing? and/or start doing?

Personal Growth Initiative: Habits of Mind

Adult Evaluation

1. Did you enjoy your involvement in this activity? Why or Why not?

2. Do you feel the student met his/her overall project goal? Why or Why not?

3. Any suggestions for the student on how his/her project could have been more successful?

4. Can you name any personal attributes or demonstrated behaviors that lead to his/her success?

Thank you for your time and effort in making this project possible!
Please sign below to verify the completion of this project evaluation.

Signature: ____

Print Name: ____

Personal Growth Initiative: Habits of Mind Grading Sheet

STUDENT NAME: ______________________ PERIOD:___ DATE:____

ORAL PRESENTATION

RUBRIC AND POINT EARNINGS

AREA	AWESOME	ACCEPTABLE	MINIMAL	UNACCEPTABLE
Content	Clearly overviewed project, reason for choosing it, and progress toward the project's goal	Described project and goal	Some explanation of project	Little to no project description
Delivery	Clear voice, loud, and pleasant Showed confidence, comfort and high degree of understanding. and preparation	Adequate voice tone and volume Appeared confident and prepared.	Low voice quality and showed little confidence and effort.	Voice tone or volume took away from delivery. Showed little to no evidence of preparation
	(15-20 points)	(10-15 points)	(5-10 points)	(0-5 points)

ORAL PRESENTATION = _____ POINTS

VISUAL PRESENTATION= _____ POINTS

TOTAL POINTS= _____

FINAL GRADE=

Personal Growth Initiative: Habits of Mind Grading Sheet Pg.2

VISUAL PRESENTATION

POSTER RUBRIC AND POINT EARNINGS

AREA	AWESOME	ACCEPTABLE	MINIMAL	UNACCEPTABLE
Content	Well-written labels captions that illustrate and inform about the meaningful project, application of the Habits and impact on personal wellness. (50-60 points)	Captions that inform viewer about the project, the 7 Habits and impact on wellness. (40-50 points)	Captions inform minimally or are incomplete about the required topics. (30-40 points)	Text is non-existent, incomplete, inaccurate, or or fail to inform (0-30 points)
Design	Layout contains appropriate photos or visuals that are easily read, logical and neat. (8-10 points)	Layout contains photos, is mostly neat, fairly logical and easy to understand . (6-8 points)	Somewhat disorganized; and hard to understand. (4-6 points)	Disorganized; appears unplanned and done hastily. (1-3 points)
Visual	Visuals capture viewer's attention and interest and are effective. (4-5 points)	Good use of color and eye-catching elements (3-4 points)	Some good ideas but something detracts from the message. (2-3 points)	Color, photos or graphic details minimal or poorly done. (1-2 points)
Creativity	Unique ideas, and/or design making the poster stand-out. (4-5 points)	Contains some unique, original, or imaginative ideas. (3-4 points)	Shows evidence of some creativity. (2-3 points)	Little or no evidence of creativity. (1-2 points)

Part Four: Selling the Program

Chapter 10: Justification

These types of programs should just sell themselves but it is not always that easy. Some key components that sell this program are how easy it is to incorporate into existing frameworks either during or after school, it takes no funding or resources (other than a willing supervisor), and satisfies many educational objectives. What I found during my recent coursework that Personal Growth Initiative can also support so many educational concepts and theories. For example, Piaget's Developmental Theory could be cited to help justify the use of this program with middle school aged students. I have had people say things like "your students are more advanced than mine to be able to accomplish those things" or "this project is above the abilities of my middle schoolers". Piaget states, the child's cognitive structures at the ages of eleven to fifteen are like that of an adult with regard to conceptual reasoning. My students have proven to me over and over again no matter where they fall on an intellectual or social continuum they are ready to take an active role in their personal growth and development. And I charge as educators that it is our duty to give them opportunities to do so.

You can use Bloom's Taxonomy of Cognitive Objectives to support this claim that these P.G.I. frameworks utilize simple to higher level thinking. Throughout this project students are asked to address all levels of the thinking hierarchy. The diagram below could be used to validate your point because it illustrates the key words, verbs and work product associated with each tier. In a P.G.I. students need to learn the concepts and demonstrate comprehension before beginning their activity (Recall & Understanding) and again during the assessment phase. They meet the objective of Application and Analysis when they develop their goals and plans. During the activity phase there could be an overlap of many skills dependant upon the situation, Application, Analysis, Synthesis and Evaluation will come into play. The personal reflection aspect of the assessment directly supports the evaluation objective.

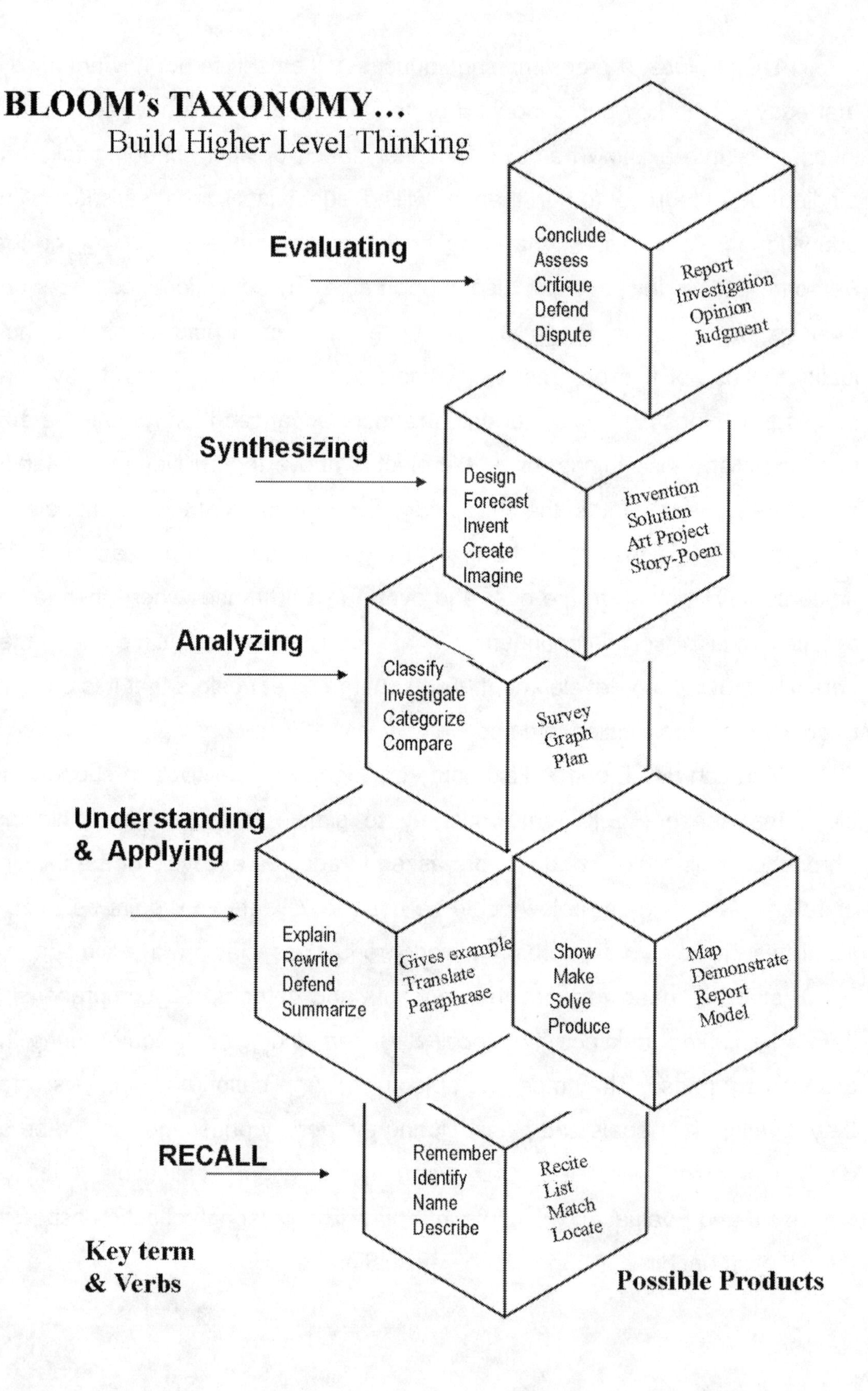
BLOOM's TAXONOMY…
Build Higher Level Thinking
Evaluating
Conclude
Assess
Critique
Defend
Dispute
Report
Investigation
Opinion
Judgment
Synthesizing
Design
Forecast
Invent
Create
Imagine
Invention
Solution
Art Project
Story-Poem
Analyzing
Classify
Investigate
Categorize
Compare
Survey
Graph
Plan
Understanding
& Applying
Explain
Rewrite
Defend
Summarize
Gives example
Translate
Paraphrase
Show
Make
Solve
Produce
Map
Demonstrate
Report
Model
RECALL
Remember
Identify
Name
Describe
Recite
List
Match
Locate
Key term
& Verbs
Possible Products

I could also give you cause to throw around educational jargon like; "differentiated learning", "student-centered" and "student driven" because a P.G.I. exemplifies each of them and it is philosophical in tune with theories like Multiple Intelligences and William Glasser's Choice Theory. A P.G.I. is by definition student centered and driven with the teacher's role as supervisor and consultant. As I have said before this approach is imperative not only for them to achieve genuine personal growth, but results in higher engagement, motivation, productivity, achievement and sense of self-competence. It can be said that this approach is the complete opposite of "one size fits all". By its design, working as an individual on a project suited to your values and concerns allows the student to utilize different learning styles and tap into multiple intelligences. Students are able to choose not only their own content and process but have quite a bit of flexibility when it comes to their evaluation tool (poster) which allows for varying abilities and types of expression. Where some students get very visually creative, others use more of the written word to convey information about their projects on their final posters.

Another selling point is that there is very little need to adapt this project to the needs of lower functioning students because each student has the ability to create the project that best suit him/her. These students like not feeling "singled out". I believe just the fact that my special education students know that they are doing the same project that all the other students are doing empowers them. Though I use modified handouts and project packets with some of my students they are unaware because it looks just like the "regular" packet (these materials can be found in Chapter 6).

Where as human nature would dictate it is typical for students to choose activities that utilize their known strengths in a P.G.I. they are often faced with having to tap into lesser used styles and intelligences. In the diagram, I have listed some of the specific skills of each intelligence area that can be practiced in a Personal Growth Initiatives.

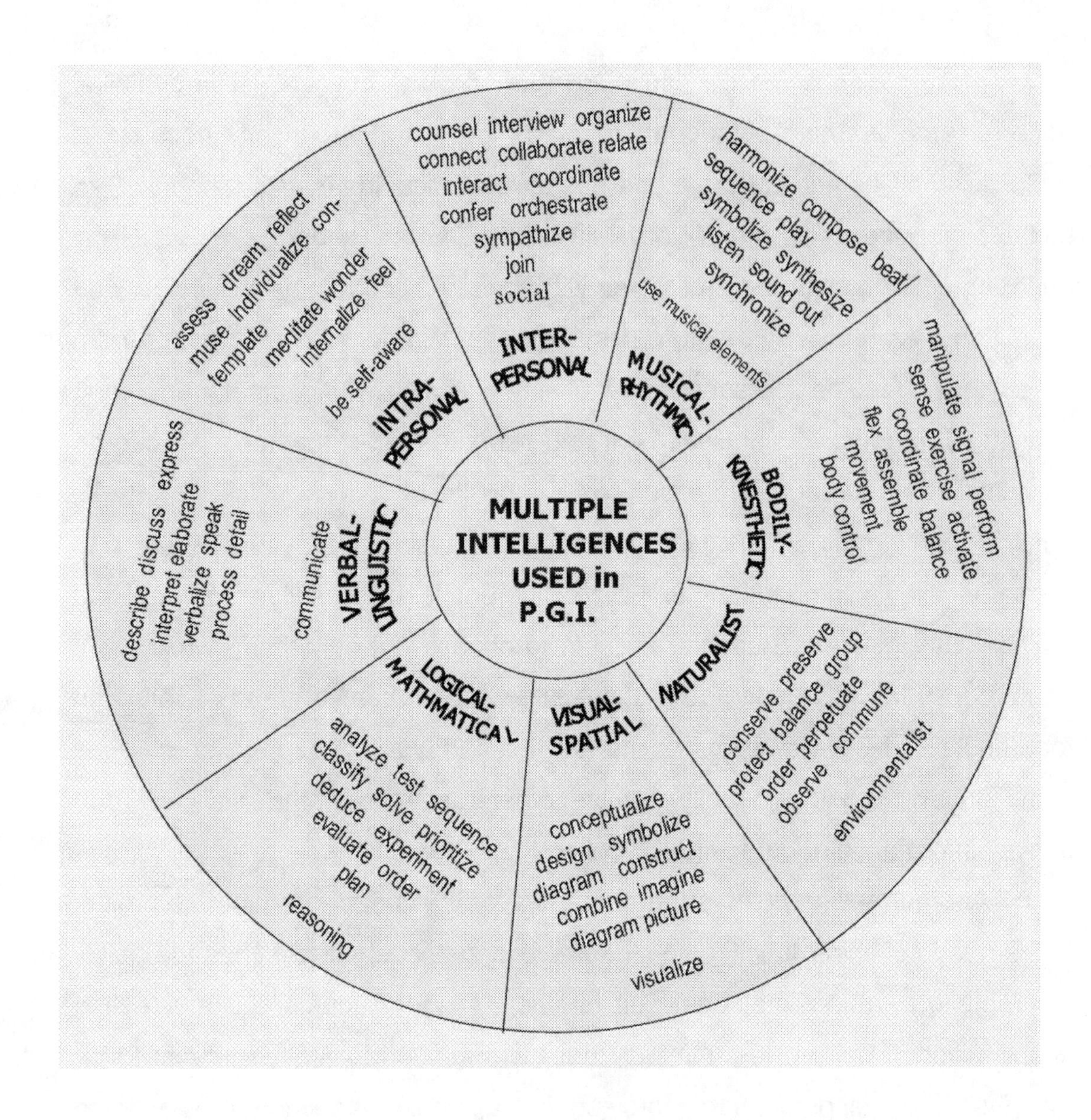

If you are not familiar with William Glasser's book titled Choice Theory or his theory which is often called "Control Theory", I will cover it more detailed in Chapter 9. For the purposes of justifying this program, his theory revolves around what he sees as the four basic needs of humans; gaining power, being free, belonging and having fun. Educationally speaking that means in order for students to value learning and take on responsibilities they need to feel that the process is in some way fulfilling their basic needs and connected to their vision of "a good life". P.G.I. should support their vision of a good life because their activity goals originate from their own concerns and values and their autonomy during the project taps into their want for power and freedom. The amount of feeding of one's need for belonging is dependent upon each student's particular activity choice, however at the conclusion everyone shares their poster and experience with their classmates to fulfill that need as well.

If you are a Health educator, a P.G.I. should be an easy sell! The use of the HEAP (CCSSO Health Education Assessment Project) framework based upon the National Standards for Health Education and terminology can clearly show how this type of project promotes each quality of a health literate person. The standards fall into eight categories and they are: Core Concepts, Assessing Information, Self-Management, Analyzing Influences, Interpersonal Communication, Decision Making, Goal Setting and Advocacy. The chart below demonstrates how often each Health Standard is addressed while the participants work at practicing the 7 Habits of Highly Effective people.

	The 7 Habits of Highly Effective People						
Health Standards	Be Proactive	Begin with the End In Mind	Put First Things First	Think Win-Win	Seek First to Understand, Then to be Understood	Synergize	Sharpen the Saw
Core Concepts	X			X	X	X	
Assessing Information		X	X		X	X	
Self-Management		X	X	X			
Analyzing Influences		X	X	X	X	X	X
Interpersonal Communication	X	X		X	X	X	
Decision Making	X	X	X	X	X	X	
Goal Setting	X	X	X		X		X
Advocacy	X	X			X		X

The following pages describe in detail how each standard can be addressed while using the 7 Habits of Highly Effective People in a P.G.I. Please feel free to use these pages to help you justify using P.G.I. in Health Education.

CORE CONCEPTS

HEALTH EDUCATION STANDARD 1: Students will comprehend concepts related to health promotion and disease prevention.

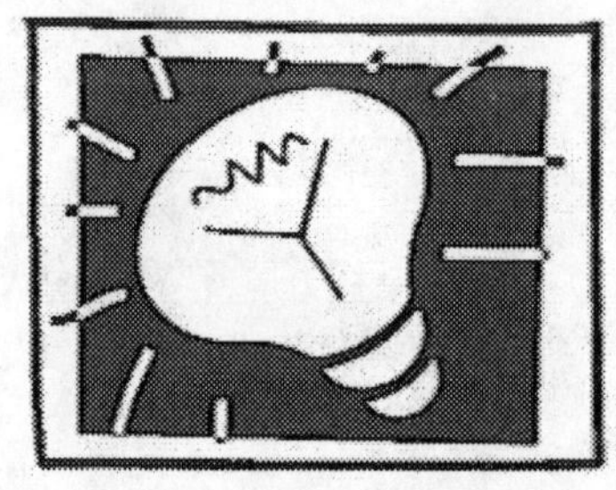

PROJECT GOALS

1. Identify the concepts utilized to promote health and/or prevent unhealthy behaviors.
2. Show relationships among ideas and concepts.
3. Make conclusions about accuracy of information.

ACCESSING INFORMATION

HEALTH EDUCATION STANDARD 2: Students will demonstrate the ability to access valid health information and health-promoting products and services.

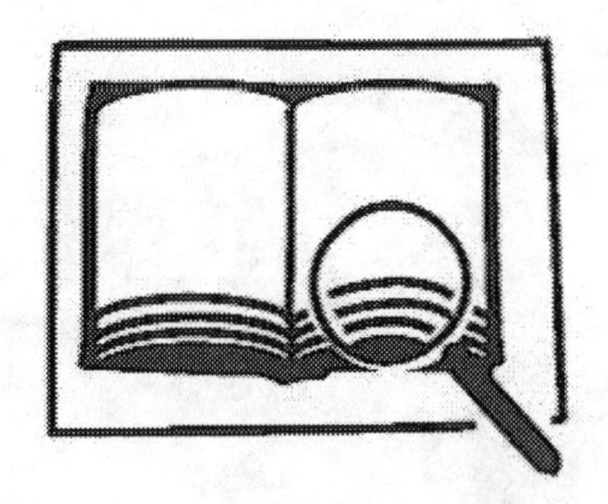

PROJECT GOALS

1. Identify sources of information and resources.

2. Analyze how sources impact project's success.

SELF MANAGEMENT

HEALTH EDUCATION STANDARD 3: Students will demonstrate the ability to practice health enhancing behaviors and reduce health risks

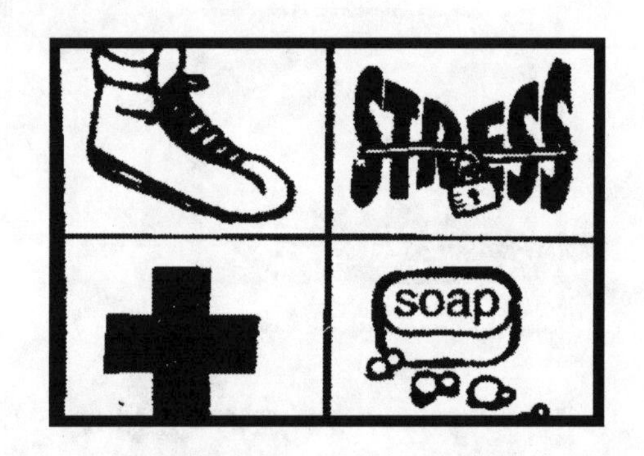

PROJECT GOALS

1. Demonstrate habits that contribute to health.

2. Explain how steps taken have improved health.

ANALYZING INFLUENCES

HEALTH EDUCATION STANDARD 4: Students will analyze the influence of culture, media, technology, and other facts on health.

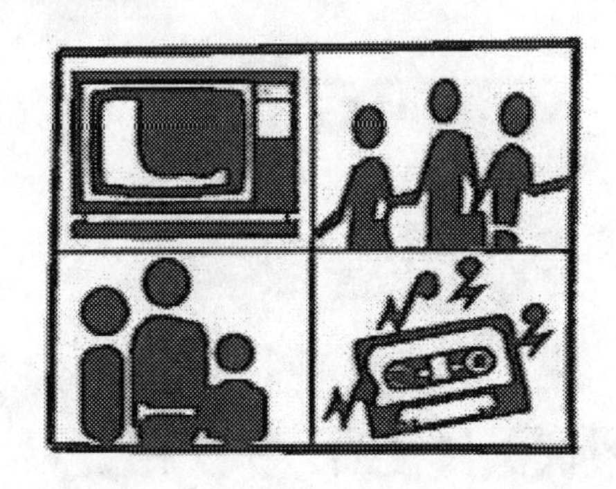

PROJECT GOALS

1. Identify internal and external influences that contributed to project's success.

2. Explain about influences that may affect future health behaviors.

INTERPERSONAL COMMUNICATION

HEALTH EDUCATION STANDARD 5:
Students will demonstrate the ability to use interpersonal comunication skills to enhance health.

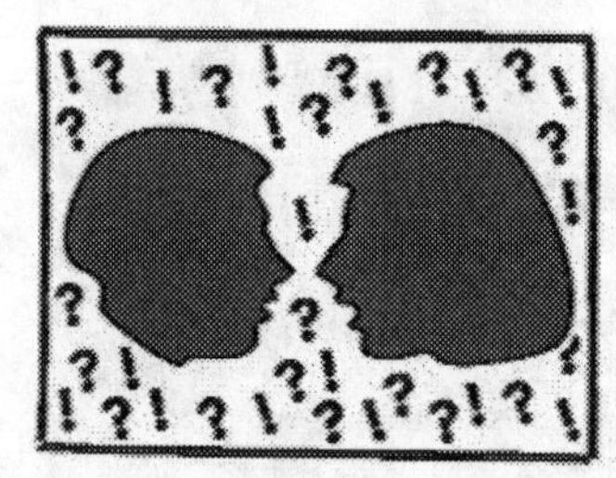

PROJECT GOALS

1. Demonstrate ability to actively listen for content and meaning.

2. Demonstrate ability to clearly express ideas and needs.

3. Analyze how communication

DECISION MAKING

HEALTH EDUCATION STANDARD 6:
Students will demonstrate the ability to use goal-setting and decision making skills to enhance health.

PROJECT GOALS

1. **Identify options and possibilities that were considered.**

2. **Identify the decisions made.**

3. **Evaluate how the decisions impacted the outcome.**

GOAL SETTING

HEALTH EDUCATION STANDARD 6: Students will demonstrate the ability to use goal-setting and decision making skills to enhance health.

PROJECT GOALS

1. Create goal(s).

2. Design a plan to meet goal(s).

3. Demonstrate how to evaluate and adjust plan if needed.

ADVOCACY

HEALTH EDUCATION STANDARD 7:
Students will demonstrate the ability to advocate for personal, family and community health.

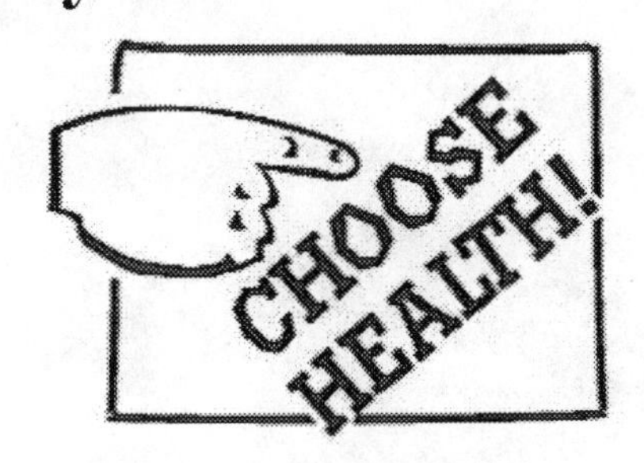

PROJECT GOALS

1. **Create a meaningful goal based on values and concerns.**

2. **Reflect upon personal growth and impact on others.**

3. **Share goals and project experience with others.**

Chapter 11: Publicity

I am lucky to have supportive administrators and colleagues. Often they become involved in student projects in one way or another. Many of the project activities are performed in our building and without the support of staff would be far less successful. The staff appreciates how these activities foster the building environment as a whole and are often fun too. If a project is being done during the school day or in the building, students are required to have a sit down meeting with an administrator for approval. If you are lucky to have willing and able administrators, as I am, this has proven to prevent miscommunication and many other problems. Also, when students are asked to sit down with the Principal, Assistant Principal or Dean it shows them that the P.G.I. is part of our school community. The support and involvement by the entire school community has evolved as the project has over the years.

Publicity Tools to Utilize:

1. **Bulletin Boards**
2. **In-School Announcements or Daily Bulletin**
3. **Student newspaper articles**
4. **PTA / Parent Newsletter announcements**
5. **Local Newspapers articles and photos**
6. **Local television stations coverage Presentations to parents and faculty: Open Houses, Faculty meetings**

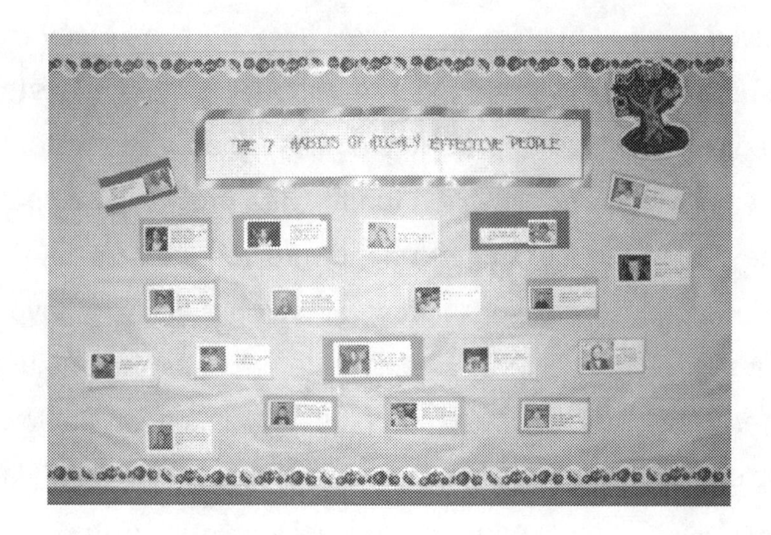

How you choose to start out should be based upon knowing your personal situation and personality, you might want to start small and quietly or with a unified large communal effort. Our program started out as a little known long term project assignment in the Health classes. As we shared student work, their posters and achievements at Open House nights with parents and with faculty at faculty meetings the appreciation and support of the potential of this project grew. Articles are placed from time to time in the student newspaper and in the parents' newsletter. Students have also tapped into these two resources as opportunities to enlist support of their projects. Our students have been given the opportunity to use the morning and afternoon announcements to further help reach their goals. I also have made bulletin boards with the students' final posters and postings of individual project ideas in progress throughout the year. This attracts attention of the students and visitors to the building. Last year, many of our students' posters were displaced in the Central Office Building outside the superintendents' offices.

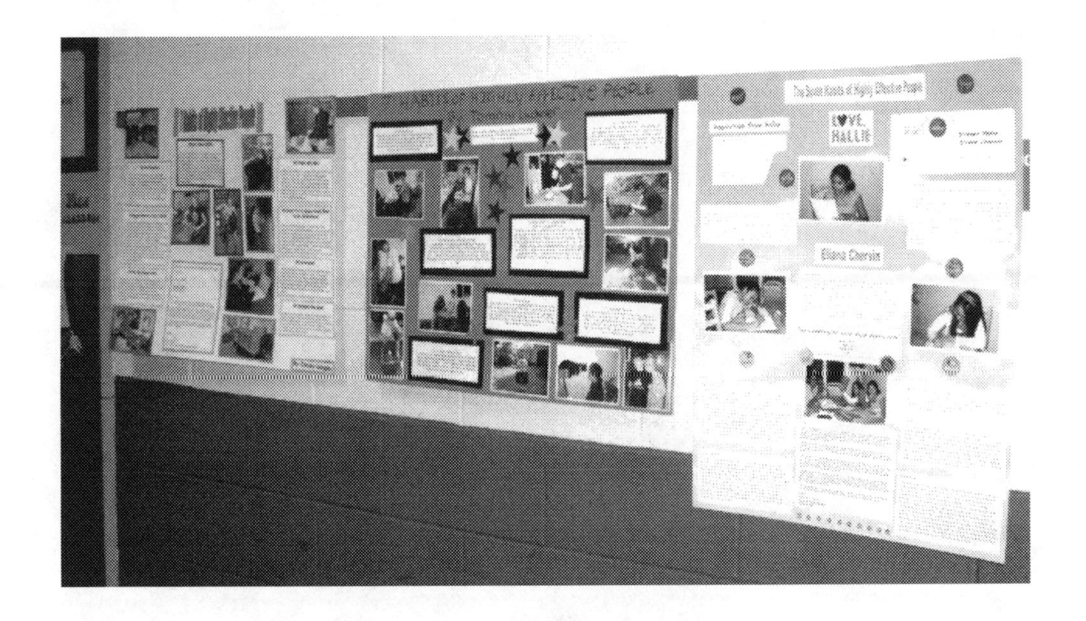

Many of these projects have been media-worthy stories that have attracted reporters from local papers and television. The attention students received was wonderful for those individuals but also in promotion of the P.G.I. as a whole. The fact that people around town know about the program raises the level of importance it has in the eyes of the participants and future participants. It also can be helpful when students ask for support or wish to offer their services out in the community. You could call the local newspaper that covers school and youth stories in your area and ask them to highlight a few of your students to get the ball rolling. Be sure to ask them to send a photographer; pictures are what catch the readers attention and the students love to see their picture in the paper.

*All articles on the following pages are reprinted with permission from the Fairfield Citizen Newspaper and Fairfield Minuteman.

'Effective' middle schoolers help others

BY ANDY HUTCHISON

Whether it's finding families for homeless dogs or providing entertainment to the elderly, Fairfield Woods Middle School seventh-graders have helped make the world a better place for many others during this school year.

Following some advice from Stephen R. Covey's book "The 7 Habits of Highly Effective People," students took on projects that gave them a taste of freedom and gave others opportunities they might not otherwise have. The students had six to eight weeks to plan and accomplish their projects in the fall and into the winter months.

The projects are ideal for these 11 and 12-year-olds, teacher Cathy Hamill said. "When they start to get into seventh grade, it's part of their personality. They're ready to step into something more independent.

"It's one of the first times they take a step forward on their own. It encourages independence in a positive way," Hamill said of the projects.

This year, over 200 students in Hamill's and Tina Bengermino's health classes picked their own ways of helping others, then followed the seven habits from the book, which include being proactive, thinking "win/win" and seeking first to understand then be understood.

Marisa Rivera and Lauren Hewitt went to Fairfield's animal shelter and put together flyers advertising the various breeds of dogs that need homes. They took pictures of the animals and wrote information such as gender, breed and age to promote the animals. After stuffing mailboxes in their neighborhoods and hanging posters on the walls at school, Rivera and Hewitt had some success.

"They did have a dog adopted as a result of this," Hamill noted.

"That was our goal — to get at least one dog adopted," Marisa said. "Animals are a big part of my life," said Lauren, who has six pets at home.

Marissa Dick went to the Jewish Home for the Elderly where her dog, "Misty", happens to work. "My dog is a therapy dog there," Marissa explained. She took pictures of "Misty" with the people at the elderly home to give to them. "My dog loves it. I think it's fun, too," she said.

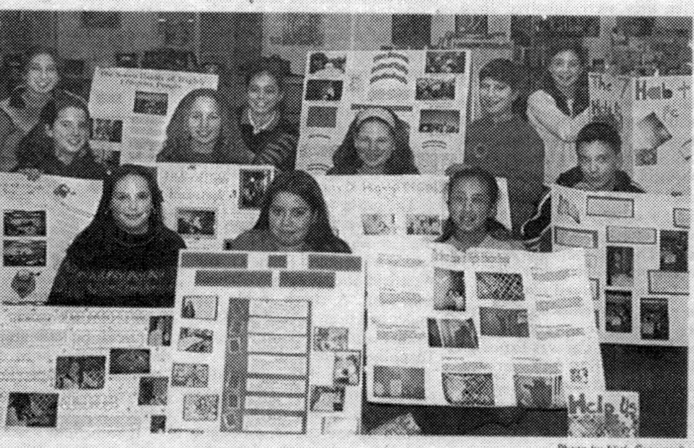

Photo by Nick Capozzoli

Helping hands on display

Fairfield Woods seventh graders spent this fall and winter planning and implementing community projects outlined on their posters.
From left, first row: Danielle Pulton, Molly Bisceglia, Marissa Rivera;
second row: Lauren McAuliffe, Marissa Dick, Stephanie Raddock, David DeBernardis;
third row: Annie Rosenblum, Caroline Ferrante, Matt Scinto, and Lauren Hewitt.

Going door-to-door, Matt Scinto raised $250 for diabetes research and participated in the Walk For Diabetes at Jennings Beach in the fall. Following "Habit 4," which is to "Think Win-Win," Scinto handed out fact sheets to those who did not donate so that they would understand how diabetes effects people.

Some of the projects brought students out of town and into neighboring Bridgeport.

Stephanie Raddock worked with her sister's Girl Scout troop to collect items for women and girls to bring to the Bridgeport Rescue Mission. "It was fun to work with the Girl Scouts and help do things for less fortunate people," she said.

David DeBernardis donated toys to the Boys and Girls Village in Bridgeport after spending a couple of hours collecting donations from customers at Kay-Bee Toys.

"It was fun to see the kids get so happy over one single toy," DeBernardis said.

Each student made a poster which explained ways they used the "7 Habits." DeBernardis followed Habit 6: "Synergize" by taking into consideration the ideas of others to collect toys. "I would have never been able to accomplish goals for this project if I didn't use other people's suggestions," he wrote on the poster.

Molly Bisceglia attended a first grade class and made "holiday hangers" with the younger students. The first-graders, whom Molly said brought her back in time, pasted their pictures on design

See STUDENTS, Page A8

Environmental Endeavor

Seventh-Grader Leads FWMS Recycling Effort

BY ALEXIS P. HARRISON
aharrison@bcnnew.com

When Aine O'Sullivan began her project for health class in March on the Seven Habits of Highly Effective People, she never envisioned the entire school would become involved or that a local business would recognize her efforts.

As part of the seventh-grade health curriculum at Fairfield Woods Middle School, students have to incorporate Stephen Covey's Seven Habits of Highly Effective People into a project and give to the class a visual and verbal presentation of how they used the seven habits. The seven habits include: be proactive; begin with the end in mind; put first things first; think win-win; seek first to understand, then to be understood; synergize; and sharpen the saw – meaning, reflection.

Aine recycled paper throughout the entire school for one week. She distributed garbage bags to each class and encouraged the classes by displaying posters with facts about recycling and the dangers if people don't recycle.

One startling fact she educated her peers on is that each day people generate 4.5 pounds of garbage. At the end of the week, she and some helpers collected all the bags of paper and weighed them, sorted the paper and loaded the bags into her father Patrick's car. Then he brought the paper to the town dump — all 2,641 pounds of it.

"We were really surprised on how much paper we collected," Aine said. She also was equally amazed how her peers took action and became as enthusiastic as she. Aine's awareness of recycling and being conscious of how humans affect the environment stems from her family. They use only organic products, everything from tin foil and paper to cans and bottles gets recycled, and paper towels are a no-no. "We are pretty committed," she said. "My mother is an environmentalist, my sister is a member of Earth Action Club at Fairfield High School and my little sister helps out."

Last week, Oliver's Nursery donated a crab apple tree to the homeroom that collected the most paper, and the tree was planted in the front of the school. "I felt very excited and proud that someone was willing to donate a tree because of a good cause," said Aine.

On Saturday, Aine participated at the Earth Day Fair hosted by the Fairfield Partnership for a Healthy Environment at Osborn Hill School. There, various vendors demonstrated how to save energy and improve the environment. Aine was in the student room and presented her project to onlookers.

Health teacher Tina Bengermino is proud of her student. "We thought it was going to be this little project, and the school took off on it," said Bengermino. "They were extremely enthusiastic and the kids really got into it."

Bengermino also applauded Oliver's generous donation to the school — which forever will capture O'Sullivan's paper drive and the students who helped make it into a reality.

Through her endeavor, Aine learned a great lesson that people do care.

"But someone has to take the first action to make them realize that they care."

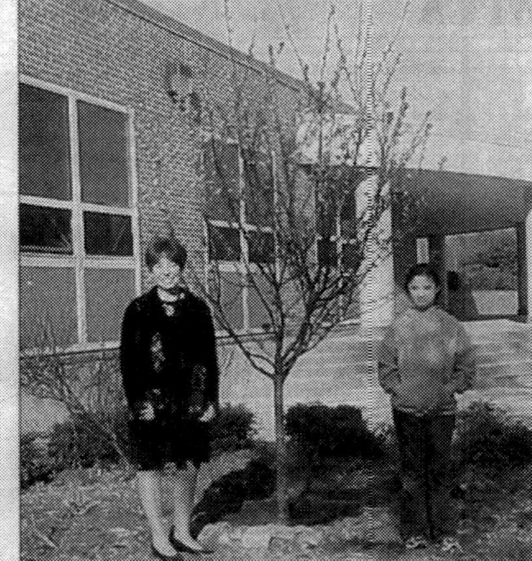

Contributed photo

A TREE GROWS AT WOODS
Fairfield Woods Middle School Principal Lynda Cox and student Aine O'Sullivan stand proudly beside the crab apple tree donated by Oliver's Nursery.

Southport Shellfish Beds Closed Indefinitely

Shellfishermen who frequent beds in Southport will have to go elsewhere for the time being.

Sands Cleary, a sanitarian for the Health Department, said yesterday that the state Department of Aquaculture has closed the shellfish beds at Southport Beach indefinitely due to tests that repeatedly resulted in high bacteria counts. Cleary could not estimate when the beds would open again.

After heavy rainfall, it is standard operating procedure for shellfish beds to be shut down for several days due to an increase in bacteria that inevitably follows. But the continual high counts "put [Southport Beach] over the edge," Cleary said.

The beds have been closed for at least several months, though all others in town remain open, he said.

Shellfish permits can be purchased through the Conservation Department at the Honorable John J. Sullivan Independence Hall; Poster's Hardware, 2155 Black Rock Turnpike; and Village Hardware, 330 Pequot Ave., Southport.

—Marc van der Pol

Student Calling All Cell Phone Owners

BY HOLLY M. PULLANO
hpullano@bonnew.com

If you have one or more "gently used" cell phones that you no longer need, Caitlin McGrath, a seventh-grade student at Fairfield Woods Middle School, hopes that you will consider donating them to her to benefit The Center for Women and Families of Eastern Fairfield County.

Caitlin is running the cell phone donation drive as part of a school health project aimed at teaching middle school students personal growth skills. For Caitlin, helping victims of domestic violence is something that she feels strongly about, which is why she chose the center as the beneficiary of her project.

According to Caitlin, she initially got the idea to collect cell phones from her older sister, who was a member of the Domestic Violence Awareness Club at Fairfield Warde High School. "The center hands out the cell phones to battered women so they can be hidden on their bodies so they can make 9-1-1 calls," Caitlin said.

Sarah Smith Lubarsky, a development associate for the center, said all types of cell phones will be accepted. Smaller cell phones will be used so that clients can keep them on their bodies to make calls in an emergency situation, while larger phones are given to a company called Pager Wizard, which exchanges the phones for money that goes into the center's client crisis service funding.

Caitlin said that while her project does not count for community service credit, it is still important for her to perform a service to the public through her health project.

Lubarsky said she is thrilled that Caitlin has chosen to help domestic violence victims and encourages the community to get involved in the project. "We think that it's wonderful for kids to be involved in service opportunities, and it's also great because it brings our services to the forefront and creates awareness of what we offer to our clients," Lubarsky said.

Tina Bengermino, Caitlin's health education teacher, was also impressed that Caitlin had taken the initiative to seek out the media in order to publicize her drive in the hopes of getting more cell phones to those who could really use them. "Caitlin has chosen to do a very worthwhile community service-type project that she is obviously passionate about," Bengermino said.

According to Bengermino, the health project itself is based on the "Seven Habits of Highly Effective

continued on page 6

FAIRFIELD CITIZEN–NEWS photo / Johnathon Henninger

Caitlin McGrath, 12, a seventh-grader at Fairfield Woods Middle School with five of the many cell phones she's collecting for The Center for Women and Families to be given to domestic violence victims.

Business Expo Today

The Regional Business Networking Expo will take place today at Norwalk Community College, 188 Richards Ave., Norwalk, from 3 to 6:30 p.m.

The event is sponsored by the Bridgeport Regional Business Council and the chambers of commerce of Darien, Fairfield, Norwalk, Westport and Stamford.

The expo and Business After Hours brings together the regional business community for networking on a grand scale and features more than 100 businesses showcasing their products.

Food and wine are available and admission is free.

IMPERATURES
r February 7:
18 H 30
low.
rise 6:58 a.m. Sunset 5:17 p.m.

TIDES
Tides at Bridgeport Harbor for February 7-12:

Fri L 9:20am	H 2:58am	Mon L 12:03pm	H 5:27am
Sat L 10:11am	H 3:44am	Tue L 1:00pm	H 6:24am
Sun L 11:05am	H 4:33am	Wed L 1:55pm	H 7:21am

2nd front

Students Learn to be Effective People

Y ALEXIS P. HARRISON
harrison@bcnnew.com

The greatest lessons in life aren't always aught in school, but for several seventh-raders at Fairfield Woods Middle School, lesson of a lifetime was not only learned ut passed on to others.

In Cathleen Hamill and Tina Bengernino's seventh-grade health classes, hands-n education is the approach and the les-on, Stephen Covey's Seven Habits of Highly Effective People. The students took he habits and conveyed them into service rojects.

"Every student was required to choose any project that they want that will enable to exercise the seven habits of highly effective people," said Hamill. "They had a six-to eight-week time period to initiate the idea and to engage in the habit until the project was complete."

After students completed the task, they presented to the class a visual and verbal attempt of how they used the seven habits. The seven habits they had to incorporate were: be proactive; begin with the end in mind; put first things first; think win-win; seek first to understand then to be understood; synergize; and sharpen the saw, meaning reflection.

The students not only had to conceptualize an idea and put it into action, but they also had to set goals for the project, have a supervising adult and plan a timeframe for

Will Grathwohl: Crafting jewelry to benefit Cancer Society

Twelve-year-old Will Grathwohl has enjoyed the Japanese art of origami or paper folding since he was four-years-old. Now the seventh-grader at Fairfield Woods Middle School, has turned his hobby into a fundraising project. Will makes origami earrings in the shape of cranes, and sells them for the benefit of the American Cancer Society.

"I've been doing origami almost all my life," Will said. "I thought this was a good idea because cranes are what you think of when you think of origami."

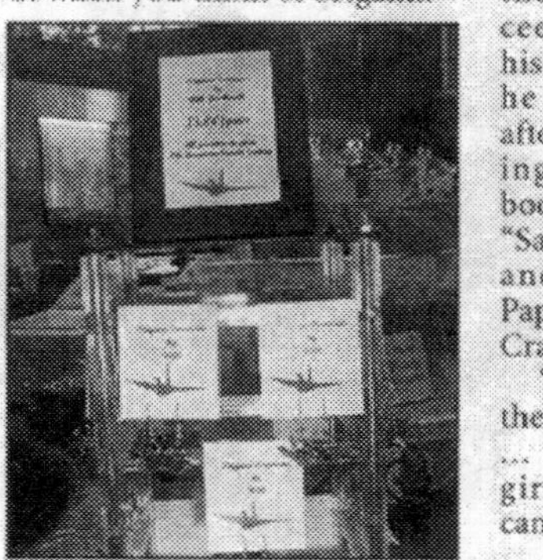

Will hand-folds each individual crane using colorful origami paper, and sprays them with lacquer to stiffen and preserve the folded paper. After they are dry, he assembles them into an earring with beads and wire. He has sold more than 30 pairs, mostly at the Chef's Table, 1561 Post Road. He sells them for $5 per pair and has already sent a check to the American Cancer Society.

Will chose that organization for the proceeds of his work, he said, after reading the book "Sadako and the Paper Cranes."

"In the book ... the girl has cancer. And that's why I'm giving the money for cancer," he said.

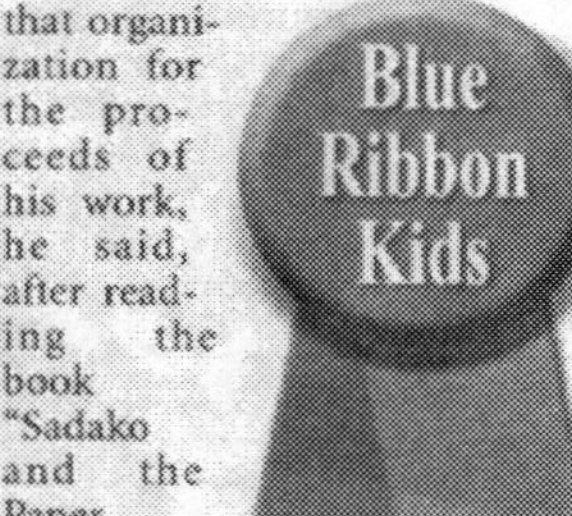

Contributed photos

Creative fundraising

Will Grathwohl presents a check to Carol Frattaroli from the American Cancer Society, money he earned by selling origami earrings he makes himself.

He will continue to make and sell the crane earrings whenever he has time, he added.

"It made me feel really good and I like helping people. It made me feel good inside and good in general."

Tomis' School Project Has Two-Pronged Effect

BY ERIN LYNCH
elynch@bcnnew.com

Vicky Tomis' school project not only helped Fairfield Animal Control, it also gave her a lesson in life.

In the early days of May Vicky, 12, was assigned a school project for her health class called Seven Habits of Highly Effective People. One of those habits includes giving back to the community. Vicky, a seventh-grader at Fairfield Woods Middle School and an animal lover, immediately thought about helping the animal shelter.

The project is based on a book of the same name written by Stephen Covey. According to Cathy Hamill, a health teacher at FWMS, the teachers use the project to teach the students basic life skills instead of giving them worksheets or tests.

Students are supposed to incorporate in their project all of the seven steps, which are to be proactive; envision their goals; prioritize; not to assume; be open to other ideas; sharpen the saw, where students should practice skills that will improve their individual growth; and think win-win, which teaches the students to tackle a situation even if they find if difficult.

For her project Vicky decided on "Coins for Cats Dimes for Dogs," in which she asked local mom-and-pop businesses if she could leave a donation can at each store, with all proceeds going toward Fairfield Animal Control.

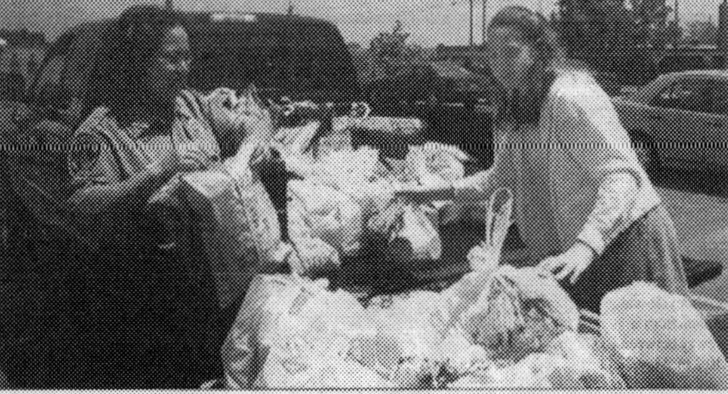

CITIZEN-NEWS photo / Erin Lynch

Animal Control Officer Rachel Solveira helps Fairfield Woods Middle School student Vicky Tomis, right, unload a truck full of goods for Fairfield Animal Control.

"One Saturday a very shy girl and her mom came to the shelter and told us about the project she wanted to do and if we would be willing to participate. I thought it was a good idea but I told her it was going to be difficult to do. But for a kid this age to go about it the way she did is very impressive," said Animal Control Officer Bill McDonagh.

After getting Animal Control's approval Vicky then approached Doughnut Inn on Black Rock Turnpike and Post Road, Lee's News Stop, The Nook, Turnpike Pet Center, The Life Gallery, Local Color, Fairfield Stationary and Bliнns, all of which agreed to be a part of her project.

Every single day Vicky went to the stores that agreed to participate in her project and collected the money. Vicky also kept a daily written and photo log of the project, which she will present during her health class on June 10.

One can was stolen from the Post Road Doughnut Inn, according to Vicky. It was returned to the store three weeks later without the money.

"I thought that I would maybe raise $200," Vicky said but after four weeks she had raised $562.01. "I didn't think I would ever get that much money, no way." Vicky said she raised $375 at the Doughnut Inn stores alone.

Vicky then took the proceeds and bought dog and cat food, leashes, collars, toys, kitten and puppy formula and bottles, bird seed, duck food, hamster food, bedding and cages, cat litter and litter pans at Pet Supplies Plus in Westport, which also supplied a 20 percent discount to Vicky. After purchasing all of the goods Vicky literally delivered a truckload of supplies to animal control on Wednesday with her mom, Debbie.

Animal Control Officer Rachel Solveira said Vicky's project "was absolutely wonderful." Solveira said she was impressed by the "time and energy" Vicky devoted to it. "It was extremely impressive how well she organized herself in collecting the money and obtaining the discount with the supplies she donated to the shelter."

Vicky said she hoped a program like her project would be offered in town. "I want the town to have a program like this one, I think it's important. This way the animal shelter could get supplies like this all the time." Vicky said she hoped various pet stores would supply donation bins so patrons could donate items that would suit animal control's needs.

According to Vicky's mom, during the project Vicky voluntarily put herself in a situation where she had to talk to people, something she doesn't normally feel comfortable with. "I'm so proud of her, our whole family is proud of her, especially because she is so shy. This was great for her self-esteem. I think this experience really helped break her out of her shell, too," Debbie said.

Vicky agrees. "This has taught me that I can really do a lot if I try harder to break out like that, it taught me that I can do anything. Because of this whole thing I feel like it made me more confident."

After delivering the supplies to the shelter on Wednesday Vicky not only came away with more confidence but she also left the shelter with a new friend, Herbie, a hamster that has been at animal control for two weeks.

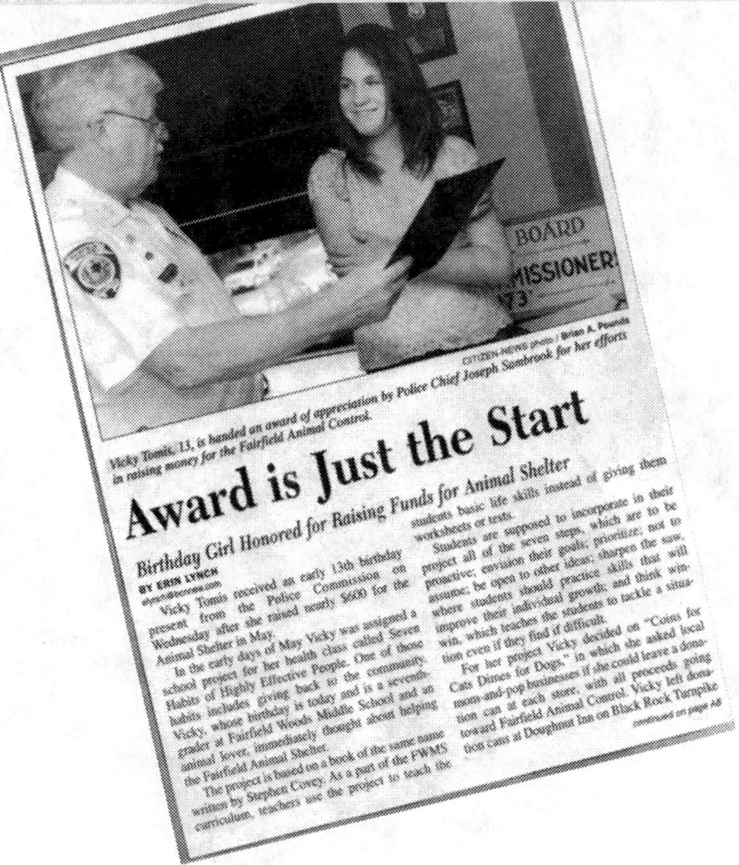

CITIZEN-NEWS photo / Brian A. Pounds

Vicky Tomis, 13, is handed an award of appreciation by Police Chief Joseph Sambrook for her efforts in raising money for the Fairfield Animal Control.

Award is Just the Start

Birthday Girl Honored for Raising Funds for Animal Shelter

BY ERIN LYNCH
elynch@bcnnew.com

Vicky Tomis received an early 13th birthday present from the Police Commission on Wednesday after she raised nearly $600 for the Animal Shelter in May.

In the early days of May Vicky was assigned a school project for her health class called Seven Habits of Highly Effective People. One of those habits includes giving back to the community. Vicky, whose birthday is today and is a seventh-grader at Fairfield Woods Middle School and an animal lover, immediately thought about helping the Fairfield Animal Shelter.

The project is based on a book of the same name written by Stephen Covey. As a part of the FWMS curriculum, teachers use the project to teach the students basic life skills instead of giving them worksheets or tests.

Students are supposed to incorporate in their project all of the seven steps, which are to be proactive; envision their goals; prioritize; not to assume; be open to other ideas; sharpen the saw, where students should practice skills that will improve their individual growth; and think win-win, which teaches the students to tackle a situation even if they find if difficult.

For her project Vicky decided on "Coins for Cats Dimes for Dogs," in which she asked local mom-and-pop businesses if she could leave a donation can at each store, with all proceeds going toward Fairfield Animal Control. Vicky left donation cans at Doughnut Inn on Black Rock Turnpike

continued on page A8

'Blue Ribbon Kids' think of others before themselves

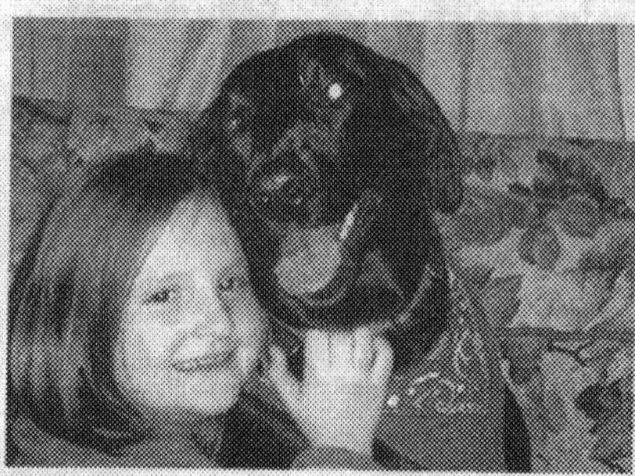

Birthday party for dogs
Megan Watts, left, had her friends donate money to the Fairfield Animal Shelter on her birthday.

Megan Watts decided to forego gifts this year for her eighth birthday. The Jennings School third grader asked her friends to donate money for the Fairfield Animal Shelter instead of buying gifts. Megan and her friends collected $321.31 for the shelter.

Megan got the idea after her family adopted several animals. They now have three dogs, a cat, a bunny, goldfish and a turtle.

"I thought that it would be nice for some animals at the shelter to get homes and get shots and have toys," Megan said. "It felt really good."

Megan brought the money to the shelter where animal control officers were very glad to get it. The reason she decided to raise the money for the shelter instead of getting her own birthday gifts was simple, according to Megan: "I really like animals," she said.

"I have four kids and all my kids love animals," said Megan's mother, Karen. "She said, 'Mom I don't need birthday gifts. Why don't I collect money for the animal shelter?'"

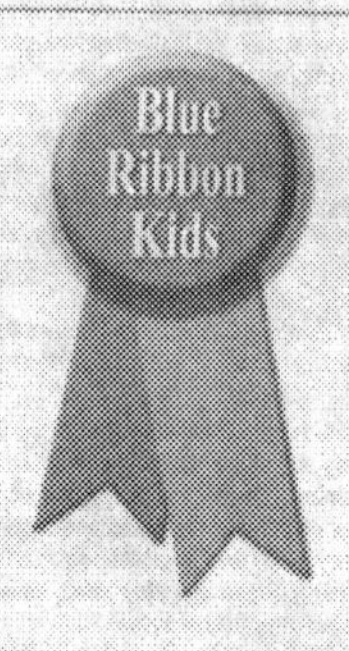

Contributed photos

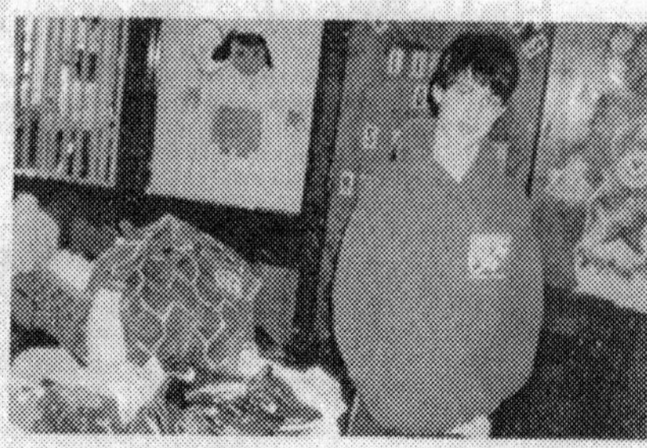

Sharing his love of soccer
Jake Blumenfeld, right, collected soccer equipment and donated it to a Bridgeport agency for children.

Jake Blumenfeld, a seventh grader at Fairfield Woods Middle School who has been playing soccer since he was four years old, donated used soccer equipment on Feb. 25 to the Charles Smith Foundation in Bridgeport.

The Charles Smith foundation sponsors programs for inner city youth and their families. The children in the program may have behavioral problems, a history of substance abuse, below grade-level reading and live in poverty.

"By donating soccer equipment, I'll be providing an opportunity for children less fortunate to have a chance to play soccer," Jake said.

Jake who has been playing on a travel soccer team for the past five years collected cleats, shin guards, uniforms and soccer balls. Since soccer has been such an important part of Jake's life, he decided this was the way to give to the community.

"I felt that I truly made a difference by donating the gently used soccer equipment," Jake said.

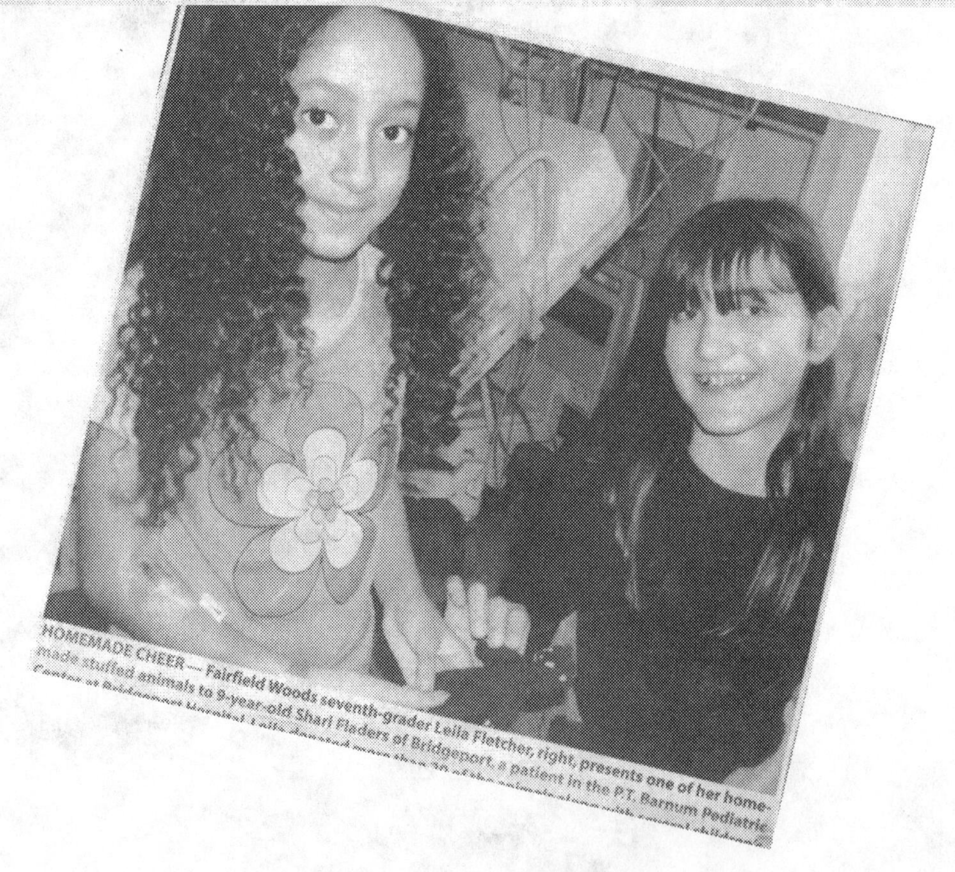

HOMEMADE CHEER — Fairfield Woods seventh-grader Leila Fletcher, right, presents one of her homemade stuffed animals to 9-year-old Shari Fladers of Bridgeport, a patient in the P.T. Barnum Pediatric Center at Bridgeport Hospital. [illegible]

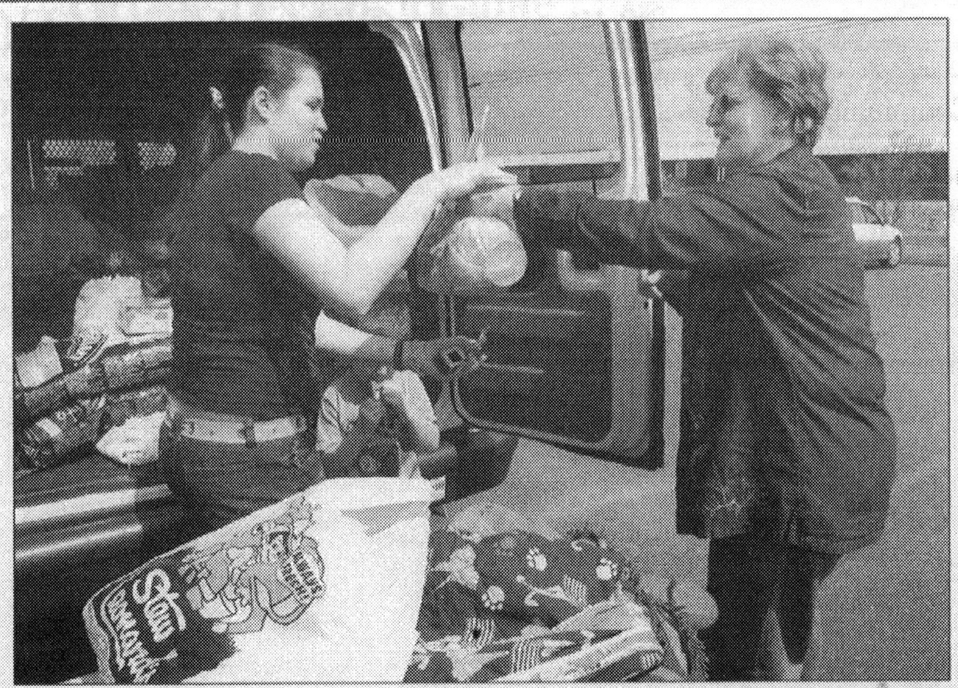

FAIRFIELD CITIZEN-NEWS photo / Tracy Deer

Help Our Pets Everyone hosted its second annual Stuff the Animal Control Van fundraiser to benefit the Fairfield Animal Shelter on Saturday. Spearheading the cause for the second year was 15-year-old Vicky Tomis, left, who accepts pet food donations from Kay Raiselis.

Residents Help Stuff the Van

BY ERIN LYNCH

elynch@bcnnew.com

Sisters Vicky and Rachel Tomis on Saturday hosted the second annual Stuff the Animal Control Van fundraiser at the Fairfield Animal Shelter, which garnered approximately $2,000 worth of donations and nearly $900 for the shelter.

The premise of the event was to invite residents to the One Rod Highway shelter with donations for the shelter such as dog and cat food and toys and try to fill the animal control van. Also, residents were invited to take part in a raffle and auction with hopes of raising money for the shelter.

Animal Control Officer Paul Miller said yesterday, "This was a fun day for everyone involved. A number of fun prizes were raffled off, and the items donated to the shelter are greatly appreciated and needed."

The raffle included gift certificates, gift baskets and sports memorabilia, including a signed football from the New England Patriots, a signed and

continued on page A8